Accident & Emergency Nursing

How to succeed and enjoy your work

Studymates

25 Key Topics in Business Studies
25 Key Topics in Human Resources
25 Key Topics in Marketing
Accident & Emergency Nursing
Business Organisation
Cultural Studies
English Legal System
European Reformation
Genetics
Macroeconomics
Organic Chemistry
Practical Drama & Theatre Arts
Revolutionary Conflicts
Social Anthropology
Social Statistics
Speaking Better French
Speaking English
Studying Chaucer
Studying History
Studying Literature
Studying Poetry
Understanding Maths
Using Information Technology

Many other titles in preparation

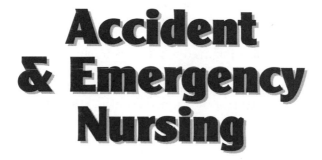

Accident & Emergency Nursing

How to succeed and enjoy your work

2nd edition

Frank Durning R.G.N.

Studymates

17.1 IHJ August 03
accident & emergency care
emergency ~~ee~~ nursing
VISA £9.99
(LC)

Notice Regarding Professional Practice

Employing organisations carry the clinical risk and vicarious liability for their employees and each practitioner is accountable for their own practice. Whether information contained in the text is applied in whole or part, the author and publishers (and any or all of their agents), emphasise that any consequence of clinical practice remains that of the healthcare professional(s) delivering clinical care. The content of this book is intended to reflect common practice within the UK at the time of writing based on the clinical experience of the author, and is written in good faith. Readers intending to use the information in the text for their practice outside the UK are reminded that differences exist in approach, terminology and drug nomenclature that could lead to misinterpretation and error. The author, the publishers and any or all of their agents cannot be held responsible or liable for the outcome of any action based on the information presented in this book, whether the professional is working within the United Kingdom or elsewhere in the world. Professionals who are in doubt over professional matters are advised to seek professional advice from more experienced colleagues.

First published in 1999 by Studymates Limited, PO Box 2, Taunton, Somerset TA3 3YE, United Kingdom

Telephone:	(01823) 432002
Fax:	(01823) 430097

Typeset by PDQ Typesetting, Newcastle-under-Lyme
Printed and bound by the Athenaeum Press Ltd, Gateshead.

1842850210

Contents

Foreword

It is with great pleasure that I write again the Foreword for the second edition of this book *Accident and Emergency Nursing* by Frank Durning. In recent times Accident and Emergency departments around the country have witnessed unprecedented pressure which is multi-factorial. Contribution made by A & E nurses is of vital importance in ensuring that the department runs smoothly and patients receive appropriate care. This has been enhanced by the NHS Plan produced by the Government, which has some brave targets to be achieved.

The role provided by A & E nurses in emergency care would further prove to be of vital importance, but that could be achieved only by understanding the subject to its fullest. As I said in my foreword for the first edition, Frank Durning's book on *Accident and Emergency Nursing* would fulfil the criteria for A & E nursing to be practical and patient orientated. The need for the second edition proves that point and I sincerely hope that the book will go from strength to strength.

G G Bodiwala, CBE, DL
DSc. (Hon.), MS, FRCS, FRCP, FFAEM, FIFEM, FICS, FICA
Accident and Emergency Department
Leicester Royal Infirmary, Leicester

March 2003

Preface

The purpose of this book is to offer practical guidance to the nurse working in an accident and emergency department within the United Kingdom, either as a student nurse on placement, or as a qualified nurse taking up a junior position within this field of nursing.

This second edition seeks to incorporate changes in practice that have evolved since the publication of the first edition. As this book is aimed at the junior nurse it is important to keep a focus on basic nursing care. The theory of more advanced practice is useful in explaining why basic care is important but it is the recognition and initial care of the A&E patient that forms the objective of this publication.

As nursing moves closer to research and evidence based practice it is important to identify those areas within accident & emergency that continue to benefit from present day research. However, this book is also a practical guide aimed at dealing with those situations for which research and academic theory may be less helpful than good examples of experiential practice that continue to yield positive results.

While it is accepted that clinical protocols will vary throughout the country depending on the designation and location of the department, it is still possible to focus on clinical practice that should be common to most establishments throughout the United Kingdom, such that a reasonable degree of uniformity can be reflected in the text.

This above all is a practical guide to the acquisition of clinical skills and practical knowledge that will give confidence to the nurse beginning as a junior member of a team within a very acute and exciting field of nursing.

The book is arranged in such a way that injuries are largely confined to anatomical areas for trauma. A separate section covers multiple injuries, cardiac arrest and procedures in the resuscitation room. The clinical specialities for which emergencies arise are also divided into individual sections for easy reference, with a separate section dedicated to paediatrics.

The field of accident and emergency nursing is both challenging and rewarding and it is the purpose of this book to provide the junior nurse with the resources for practical survival in an area of great diversity.

Frank Durning

Orientation

One-minute summary – The keys to a good orientation are mentorship, geographical knowledge and communications skills. Getting to know where the fire and clinical alarm bells are located goes hand in hand with finding out how to summon help when your workload begins to get difficult. Appropriate use of professional relationships, and realistic clinical learning objectives, will speed your progress. Clinical supervision will help to provide a forum for discussion of professional dilemmas. Knowledge of procedures such as admission and discharge will create more time for the clinical care needed between those two points. Find out what orientation programme is available to you before setting your own learning objectives.

In this chapter you will learn:

▶ the importance of contracts and geographical logistics
▶ procedures for arrival and reporting
▶ the purpose of mentorship and preceptorship
▶ specific aspects of the code of professional conduct
▶ how to set and achieve learning objectives
▶ the importance of safety and communication
▶ the A&E team structure.

Contracts and geographical logistics

Your contract and insurance at work

In order for an NHS employee to be covered by the insurance policies of the organisation in which they work, they must have signed a contract of employment. In most cases the signing of such a contract is a formality that follows interview and written confirmation of the job offer.

It is wise to ask about signing your contract on the first day you start work. Apart from the reasons of insurance cover it is normally a requirement by Payroll that a contract of employment be signed, so failure to do so could delay payment of your salary.

Finding your way around

Geographical logistics are important when you begin a new post. So often it is the little things that cause most inconvenience and anxiety. Take the trouble to pay an informal visit to the A&E department either prior to job interview or immediately afterwards. This will highlight the geographical location of your employment. It will also help you become familiar with which entrance is used by staff and where the nearest car park is. It will also indicate how much time to leave yourself when arriving for duty.

Procedures for arrival and reporting

Get to know:

▶ where to arrive for duty

▶ how to report for the start of a shift.

Some departments ask you to sign a book to denote your attendance. Others use a roll call system or even an electronic form of time keeping using a computer. Although practices vary the main modes of handover in A&E are either from the clinical areas themselves or from a designated room where a handover to the full shift can take place.

Mentorship and preceptorship

Most departments have a system of attachment for junior staff. It may be called **mentorship, preceptorship** or **buddy system** – the title doesn't really matter. What is important is that you have a designated senior person to look after your professional activities within the A&E department, particularly at the start of your contract.

Do take time at an early stage to get to know your mentor. Be open with each other in discussing your worries and expectations.

For newly qualified nurses, preceptorship should be mandatory and rather more formal than for staff who have completed their first year after qualification. Clinical supervision is something outside the role of mentor. It is designed to embrace your professional career in the wider sense and may be provided individually or as a group. Your mentor should not be your clinical supervisor.

The code of professional conduct

At the time of writing every registered nurse, midwife and Health visitor practising in the UK is required to be registered by the statutory body responsible for the maintenance of a professional register and the provision of measures that protect the public and maintain high professional standards. 'The Nursing and Midwifery Council' is the current body in the United Kingdom.

The NMC has published numerous documents relating to professional practice which can be viewed on their web site (address at the back of this book) or obtained from:

Nursing and Midwifery Council
23 Portland Place
LONDON
WIN 3AF

The code of professional conduct is the cornerstone of the standards set for the way in which the nursing profession should conduct itself. You must acknowledge limitations in knowledge and competence in dealing with patients. The wide variety of clinical activity in A&E will present situations where limitations in your competency will arise. It can sometimes be difficult for a junior staff member to decline a request from senior staff to carry out a procedure for which you are not competent. However, the consequences of embarking on such procedures, and failing, can be very serious for the patient and for yourself.

Confidentiality

This area can be very difficult in A&E – particularly when police and legal officials are compelled to ask you for information. As a junior nurse it should not be up to you to decide whether or not clinical information should be released without consent. In the absence of a departmental written policy, you should always refer such situations to a more senior nurse.

Your learning objectives

As a nurse with little or no A&E experience, you will find yourself at the start of a learning curve. This curve will vary in steepness as the days and months go by. Your employer may have given you an orientation package which sets learning objectives for you. Also, you may have objectives of your own that you would like to see built into your learning plan.

Creating your own learning plan

In the absence of any formal learning plan you may wish to consider the objectives for learning under three headings:

1. acquisition of clinical skills
2. theoretical knowledge
3. professional and academic development.

Acquisition of clinical skills

These are the clinical procedures that you should be competent to perform by a designated point in your career. These might focus on the first six weeks and then checked again at three months, then six months, and so on.

Clinical procedures within the first six weeks might include:

▶ bandaging and strapping
▶ ECG recording
▶ setting trolleys for suturing
▶ use of available equipment for taking baseline observations
▶ techniques for undressing an injured patient safely
▶ basic life support.

Theoretical knowledge

Practical clinical skills simply become tasks unless knowledge is gained to explain the reasoning behind a procedure. Acquiring theoretical knowledge is always helpful but it is more meaningful if it can be learned in conjunction with the practical skills to which it applies.

Again, it is worth looking at a time scale for theoretical learning. The first six weeks' subjects might include:

▶ physiology of sprains and strains
▶ some general skeletal anatomy
▶ the process of wound healing
▶ classification of fractures.

Professional and academic development
Professional development involves combining clinical and theoretical knowledge. You learn to apply it in such a way that you become an active member of the nursing team, taking on work in areas of particular interest, or building links with other areas of nursing that can use the experience you have gained. To be able to work relatively unsupervised in a certain area might be your first goal in professional development. You will achieve academic development by completing recognised courses in your professional field. These could include the advanced life support course, or teaching and assessing courses.

Whatever learning objectives you decide, it is important to discuss them with your mentor. Also, make your objectives realistic. It also helps if you can develop a method of learning that suits you personally, whether this means practical observation or other methods, and whether in a group or one to one.

Keep a record of your learning in your personal profile. Review it periodically to assess your progress against plan.

Safety and communication

Health and safety at work legislation continues to receive a high profile in the workplace, and A&E is no exception. (Health & Safety At Work Act 1974.) The obligation to keep you safe does not rest only with your employer; you have a duty as well. Attend the lectures on safety required by your employer and observe the policies for health and safety in your area of work.

Four key areas of health and safety
There are four specific areas that you should seek clear guidance upon early in your employment. They are:

1. the fire procedure
2. procedures relating to management of violence and aggression
3. manual handling procedures

4. procedure to be followed after a needlestick injury.

There will also be a stated procedure to follow if you have an accident at work. Do make yourself aware of your obligations under this procedure. Effective communication is vital in A&E work. When you first begin at a new department there will be many aspects of the communication system to learn about. Eventually, many of these will become second nature to you. In the first few weeks, however, it is important to learn about key aspects of communication.

Fire communications

At an early stage you should know where the fire bells and fire escapes are located in the department. You should also know where all the internal telephones are. What number should you dial in the event of fire? Where is the assembly point for evacuation?

Using the telephone

Learn the external telephone number for the hospital, and any direct external number for the department. You may need to contact the department because you are running late for duty, or because a relative asks for a contact number for future reference.

You need to know how to contact the hospital switchboard and how to make an outside call and you also need to be aware of any features that the telephone system has, such as call diversion, or secrecy options.

Bleeps

If your hospital operates a bleep system then you need to know how to bleep somebody at any time, both routinely, and urgently. You also need to know who to bleep if there is a cardiac arrest. Many A&E departments run their own cardiac arrest procedures, but it is vital to know where help comes from in those situations.

Notice boards and duty rotas

Learn where the notice boards and duty rotas are kept. Find out where the alarm points are for clinical assistance; for example, in the resuscitation room. Make a point of noting where the oxygen and suction points are in the department and whether they are wall or cylinder driven. If it is cylinder driven then learn to locate and use the keys that open the cylinders.

Forms and notes

Written communication is important. You will have to deal with clinical notes, and day to day communication between staff members inside and outside the department. Get to know what written forms are used inside the department to communicate changes, and the outcome of staff meetings. Learn to use the written communication system effectively. Learn how the internal and external mailing system operates.

Record keeping

Nursing staff must maintain a high standard of clinical documentation. Electronic documentation and decision support software is an evolving area for patient management in primary and secondary care. You should ensure that any training needs you may have in using computerised systems are made known prior to using them.

Your own department may well have its own policy on written standards of documentation. If it does, you should read it and follow it. Acquire a blank set of notes to study clinical documentation used in your department. In some places the nursing and medical notes are combined; in others they are separated. Make sure you know what you are expected to document, especially concerning the administration of drugs.

The A&E team structure

An A&E department is a multi-disciplinary team. It works together at all levels for the common good of the patient. There are numerous components in the team. These typically include nursing and medical staff, porters, cleaners, radiographers, play specialists, clerical staff, pharmacists, clergy and social workers, in addition to external medical specialists, when required.

It is essential for all members of the team to recognise the value of everybody's contribution. Without this commitment, the flow of patients through the department would be disrupted and patients could be placed at risk. Even seemingly trivial situations can cause significant problems.

▶ *Example* – Full waste bins in the resuscitation room could quickly become a clinical hazard if cleaners were not on hand to empty them.

Suppose the clerical workers failed to produce notes for patients. It would be extremely difficult to know what treatment a patient had received. It could even result in the wrong treatment being given.

While no single individual is ever indispensable we all have our role to play within the A&E team. Let's now explore that role a little further.

Your role in the team

As a junior member of staff, your first and most obvious role as a team member is to support the senior staff as much as you can. You are helping them carry out the contractual clinical and professional duties laid down by the policies of the department.

Peer support during this time is essential. Just as you receive support from other members of junior staff, you too can lend support to those who need it. You could offer practical help with a clinical problem, or lend a listening ear when other colleagues want to talk about situations that are making them anxious.

Your department will decide which roles you can or cannot take on. Only by asking senior staff, and your mentor, will your role become clearer to you as you gain experience.

It is important that, as a member of the A&E team, you project the confidence and professionalism expected from this 'shop window' of the hospital. Someone may ask you to carry out a task that you have never done before, yet it would be a disaster to utter that fact to the patient who is likely to be far more apprehensive than you. Indeed, the role of a junior nurse within a department is in many respects more demanding than that of a senior nurse, because of situations such as that just described.

If you are not sure of how to deal with such a situation, excuse yourself from the patient. Then ask the member of staff who made the request to join you for a moment, out of the patient's earshot. You can then discuss the matter in private and gain the knowledge to do the task, or have the task assigned to somebody else.

The key to performing your role as an effective member of the A&E team rests on you. Show that you are willing to learn. Show courtesy, professionalism and regard for others. In this way others will readily relate to you, and pass on their knowledge and skills.

It is easy to misinterpret the response of a colleague who seems short with you, or aloof. Give that individual the benefit of the doubt, at least initially. That way you may not close a valuable door of information and learning that, with patience, could be opened to you.

Remember that A&E can be a very stressful environment. Even the most experienced nurses are only human.

Summary

▶ Take time to know the exact geography of where you are going to work.

▶ Identify where the parking facilities are, and where to report for duty.

▶ Make sure you sign a contract of employment. Be careful to abide by it, along with departmental policies and the NMC code of conduct.

▶ An orientation package may have been prepared for you. Whether it has or not, you need also to agree learning objectives.

▶ Learn the location of fire bells, oxygen and suction points and internal telephones.

▶ Know who to contact in cardiac arrest and how the bleep and Tannoy systems work.

Helping you learn

Progress questions

1 Name five disciplines that provide an input to the A&E department.

2. What do you need to know in relation to any tannoy system that might be in operation within the department?

3. Give two reasons why a contract of employment is important.

Seminar discussions

1. The police ask you to report the arrival of any male in his twenties who has a hand injury. They say there has been a spate of house break-ins in the locality recently. You receive a man fitting that description. He says he cut his hand on glass while washing up last night. Do you report him?

2. A police officer arrives in the department. He asks if the patient whose hand abrasion you have just dressed five minutes ago is

displaying a tattoo mark next to the wound. The office says he may be wanted for a serious sexual assault. Do you report him?

3. Why should your mentor or preceptor not be your clinical supervisor?

Practical assignments

1. Find a spatula and write down a list of the important internal, external and tannoy numbers on it.

2. Draw up a list of four or five specific points that you would like to discuss with your mentor when you next meet.

Working Under Pressure

One-minute summary – The Accident & Emergency department is 'demand led'. The workloads and case mix are unpredictable. This is appealing to some nurses, but when the demand becomes high, all nurses still need strategies to continue working safely. Stress in small doses is manageable and healthy. However, a build up of pressure will convert stress to distress, if left unrecognised and unmanaged. It can produce unpleasant symptoms leading to dysfunction. It is important for you to be able to identify the sources of stress in Accident & Emergency departments. You should know who to communicate with, and how to communicate with them, so that you are not isolated. It is also important for you to keep a sense of priority and remain objective at busy times.

In this chapter you will learn:

▶ triggers that create stress in A&E
▶ professional communication and relationships
▶ exposure to clinical and social tragedy.

Stress triggers in A&E

The common trigger points within the field of Accident & Emergency nursing fall under three main headings:

1. workload
2. professional communication and relationships
3. exposure to clinical and social tragedy.

Let's consider them in turn.

Workload
When a department is busy, there are two situations that often produce difficulties.

(a) There is a large amount of work to get through, and you feel it is within your clinical capabilities, but the volume of work seems overwhelming, and you experience great anxiety and frustration.

(b) More senior staff appear to be very busy, while you are not able to do very much. You feel inadequate because the tasks require the skill of more senior nurses.

Coping with the high workload

In some respects the high workload situation is easier to manage than lack of experience. If you are short of work, as more senior nurses become busy, then use the opportunity as a learning experience. Observe carefully, and ask questions.

Coping with a high volume workload will become easier for you when you know the following facts about the area to which you are allocated:

What are the boundaries of this area?

This may seem a rather obvious question to ask at a very early stage. But it is worth clarifying with the nurse in charge. Special working arrangements sometimes come into force when volumes are high, or when there is a change in work patterns from day to night. The nurse in charge may assign you a 'watching brief' over a relatively low dependency area, while more experienced nurses are assigned elsewhere.

Who is here to help and whom do I ask if problems arise?

At very busy times staff may have to be reallocated in order to match resources to clinical demand more effectively. You need to be clear who is working with you in a particular area, and where your immediate help will come from if problems arise.

If your source of help is working in another area, then make sure how you are going to communicate. It is far less stressful to have a pre-planned system of communication that is not used, than to suddenly require help urgently and not know where to find it.

Where are the sources of work for this area?

It is important to know where your sources of work within an area lie, and how to access them. For example:

▶ In a minor injuries area the patient notes may be first stored at triage from where you are required to call the patient round.
▶ There may be a separate box for the notes of patients awaiting treatment from you.
▶ There may be a separate arrival point for patients arriving by ambulance.

Once the sources of work are known, staff can find an appropriate method of prioritising the workload.

What are my priorities?

When you receive a handover, ask what is the first priority. Make sure you deal with that first. It is not always possible to deal with one priority, and then neatly move to another, but try to organise priorities as you see them at the time.

When several priorities seem to be arising at once, tell the nurse in charge. This may not bring you instant help, but it will reassure the nurse in charge that you are using your judgement. This in turn will increase your confidence to go on working effectively in spite of a heavy workload.

When should I ask for help?

There is an instinctive dilemma here for most nurses:

(a) On the one hand they must work within the NMC code of professional conduct. They must acknowledge limitations in skill, and highlight environments that are unsafe.

(b) On the other hand, they want to be seen to cope. They do not want to be seen to fail, or to appear unsupportive to colleagues.

The answer to this dilemma is safety. Pressure within your area is probably building up because of equal or greater pressure elsewhere. This should not affect your decision to ask for help; it should alter the way in which you ask.

If you feel that the workload within your area of responsibility is putting patient safety at potential or actual risk, then you are duty bound to make that known to the nurse in charge.

Explain that you understand that other areas are busy, too. This may help to smooth things with the nurse in charge, who may not view your problems as an immediate priority.

Your coping strategy here is based on the fact that, no matter how bad things become after you have asked for help, it is now the responsibility of the nurse in charge to initiate corrective action within your area. As a junior nurse you will have met your responsibilities. You have obtained some possibility of reducing the pressure rather than suffering in silence, and having the nurse in charge take more corrective action than might have been necessary.

Professional communication and relationships

Do I know the telephone, bleep and tannoy system well enough to communicate effectively?

Good communication is everything in Accident & Emergency. Even experienced clinicians become uneasy when it fails. A positive way you can reduce the anxiety for yourself and colleagues, when working under pressure, is to make sure you know the telephone, bleep and tannoy systems. Knowledge of these systems ensures the movement of patients through the system. Here are some helpful tips for good communication.

Note down essential numbers
Acquire a couple of spatulas, and write down essential numbers such as internal department extensions, numbers for support departments such as X ray, Fracture Clinic, Biochemistry and Haematology labs.

Using the bleep
Make sure you know how to activate a bleep for someone. Make sure you can do it both for someone you need routinely, and for someone you need in an emergency. Many bleeps work in these two modes. If you carry a bleep yourself, make sure that you know how to answer it, silence it, and change its batteries.

Understanding the tannoy
Learn the most commonly used numbers for tannoys if they are installed. Learn the verbal format that is used to make announcements. There may be **coded messages** for summoning help. These keep the nature of a call recognisable only to staff. Make sure you know how to switch a tannoy off after an announcement.

What form of address is used 'on the shop floor'
Get to know how nurses communicate with each other in the presence
of patients. It can be confusing when some units use first names, while
others use formal titles and surnames.

Find out what the professional chain of communication is for specific
situations such as:

▶ admitting a patient to a ward
▶ giving information to a relative
▶ requesting the attendance of senior medical staff
▶ dealing with a patient who wishes to take their own discharge.

Understanding these communication systems will reduce the pressure
on you at times of increased workload.

Exposure to clinical and social tragedy

Dealing with death, severe illness, injury, and social poverty, week in
week out, can be a prelude to pressure and stress. There is also the
problem of escalating violence in hospitals, as in society at large.

Coping strategies
Coping strategies for managing this type of work pressure need to be
clearly set out. It is important for you to discuss your clinical
experiences with colleagues, and with more senior staff, as soon
afterwards as you can.

Debriefing
The purpose of this 'debriefing' is:

1. to identify the thoughts and feelings that staff may have following a
    distressing incident, and

2. to evaluate the professional response to the incident, so as to
    identify possible improvements for the future.

Value of clinical knowledge
Junior nurses may experience considerable pressure as a result of
dealing with such incidents as sudden infant death or multiple trauma
in young people. This pressure largely arises from a lack of clinical
knowledge. It can distort the nurse's perception of such an event. If you

discuss the incident with somebody more experienced, your perception can sometimes end up being quite different, even though the event itself is tragic and distressing.

Putting stress into perspective

Repeated exposure to stressful situations makes it difficult for any human being to function properly. These stresses can build up quite rapidly when the workload involves dealing constantly with accidents and illness resulting from poverty, depression and dispute. Such a workload is in the very nature of a typical A&E department, but it is often difficult to keep things in proportion.

During the course of a shift you may have dealt with four or five overdoses and three or four assaults. But remember, this is not typical of the local population as a whole. As a junior nurse, your workload is – by very definition of 'accident' and 'emergency' – one of exposure to the abnormal.

Normality returns at the end of the shift. It is important for you to learn how to psychologically 'switch off' as the shift ends.

Summary

- ▶ Stress in A&E originates from problems of workload, communication, and clinical or social tragedy.
- ▶ Identify a mentor with whom you can discuss your concerns.
- ▶ Take a logical approach to creating priorities.
- ▶ Work within your own limitations. Seek help when these limits are exceeded.
- ▶ Keep a perspective – while you are dealing with a few patients in tragic circumstances, most people elsewhere are having a perfectly normal day.
- ▶ Problems that you keep taking home are the very ones that you should discuss with senior colleagues.

Helping you learn

Progress questions

1. Name three triggers that produce stress in A&E.

2. What can you contribute as a junior nurse, when most of the workload seems to be for more experienced nurses?

Seminar discussions

1. What signs would tell you that you were not coping well with the stress of A&E?

2. Your area comes under unexpectedly heavy pressure, and the nurse in charge is extremely busy elsewhere. What do you do?

Practical assignments

1. Choose a particular area within the department. Compare how it is staffed between day and night shifts.

2. Find out the total number of patients that attend the A&E department in a year. Discover how many nursing hours exist in the year to provide the service.

Assessment & Observations

One-minute summary – If a patient deteriorates thirty minutes after arrival in A&E, the only way of measuring the deterioration is to compare the original observations recorded on arrival with those now. More often than not, it is an abnormality picked up in routine baseline observations that offers the key to a diagnosis – not the complex and expensive investigations that take place further down the line. A patient's skin colour, texture, level of consciousness, and respiratory rate will provide all the evidence needed to say that a patient is sick, without even touching the patient. Baseline observations are probably the most important aspect of A&E nursing.

In this chapter you will learn:

▶ how to take an accurate history
▶ the importance of using anatomical references
▶ the relevance of previous medical history
▶ the observations required for a patient in A&E.

Taking an accurate history

A patient's history will derive from a combination of three sources:

1. the patient
2. relatives or witnesses from the scene
3. relatives or other professionals remote from the scene.

Accuracy and expediency are the essentials of good history taking. Many patients can convey their history in such a manner; others need a systematic and skilled approach in order to glean the right quality of information relevant to their attendance.

Patients without clear histories

It can reasonably be expected that three categories of patient will not tender clear histories on their own:

1. patients with an impaired level of consciousness
2. the elderly or the very young with communication impairment
3. the patient whose language cannot be understood.

In these situations the nurse must rely on a third party to provide whatever information they can. This highlights the importance of listening to those who accompany the patient to hospital, or who provide written information; such as a general practitioner or care home.

Patients able to give their history

For those patients who communicate for themselves, the taking of a history may still require some guidance. Remember, only relevant information is required.

A judgement also needs to be made as to whether the patient is safe to offer their history before any urgent intervention.

▶ *Example* – A 45 year old male presents with central crushing chest pain. He is clammy and sweaty.

Clearly this is a situation where the patient is clinically in the acute stages of a myocardial infarction. To delay physical care for the purpose of taking the history is unsafe. This patient requires a nurse who can begin clinical management while listening to the history at the same time.

Taking a good history

There are five components to taking a good history:

1. What happened?
2. How long ago did it happen?
3. What mechanism or forces were involved (if any)?
4. What are the primary symptoms?
5. Were there any previous incidents or relevant history?

This checklist can be applied to both trauma and acute illness. The same sequence of events and nature of symptoms are required for both. However, some flexibility is required for the more chronic illnesses, where the pattern of events can be long drawn out and fragmented.

What happened?
This question puts the focus on the events immediately prior to and during the accident or incident of illness.
    'I was coming downstairs and I tripped.'
    'I was working in the garage and my ankle became painful.'

How long ago did it happen?
This is a very important question. It will determine the investigation and treatment of an injury or illness based on the pathology that occurred between onset and presentation.
    'It happened 20 minutes ago.'
    'It must be about three days ago now.'

What mechanisms or forces were involved?
Speed, force, impact and direction all play a part in determining the degree and location of clinical pathology. We will come to this in more detail in other chapters.
    The range of mechanisms commonly involved in trauma include:

1.   direct blow
2.   indirect blow
3.   crush
4.   walking, running, jumping
5.   twisting, bending, stretching.

    'When I was running I tripped and my ankle twisted inwards.'
    'When I was walking I just felt pain increasing gradually in my ankle.'

What are the primary symptoms?
The emphasis here is on *primary* symptoms. The detail of lesser symptoms can be gleaned later as the examination proceeds.
    'My ankle is swollen and painful and I can't walk on it.'
    'My ankle hurts as I walk.'

Previous incidents or relevant history?
This is about any previous event or medical problem that could *directly* affect the way in which the present problem might be managed.
    'I am normally healthy and well.'
    'I broke this ankle just two months ago.'

Using anatomical references

As a junior nurse it is important to use anatomical references. These terms provide a universal language that can accurately describe pathology to a fellow health professional. That person could be standing next to you, or be 200 miles away reading your notes, or listening to your referral on the telephone.

Using anatomical references can be a slow process. However, as with any new language, you will become fluent with practise. Eventually you will save a lot of time through communicating in this way.

All terms of reference are taken from the position of a person standing straight and looking at you with their arms by their sides and their palms uppermost towards you.

Descriptive terms in anatomy

anterior	to the front
posterior	to the back
lateral	away from the midline
medial	towards the midline
superior	above
inferior	below
proximal	near to
distal	away from
middle	middle

From the descriptive terms above it is possible to draw the position of an injury to within fairly accurate landmarks. There are also descriptions available to determine the direction of a laceration or direction of the force that caused the injury.

vertical	from the top down
horizontal	in a linear plane
oblique	inclined at other than right angle
transverse	straight across
volar	on the palmar side of the hand and forearm
plantar	on the heel side of the foot
dorsal	on the opposite side to volar and plantar

The relevance of previous medical history

The A&E patient is in a different setting than that of a GP's surgery or hospital out patient department. In those environments, more time can be devoted to the detail of past medical history. However it is important in A&E to establish any history relevant to the causation of injury or illness with which the patient has presented, or to any treatment that may be carried out in A&E.

There are four main headings to note as a minimal requirement in a past medical history:

▶ allergies
▶ present prescribed and recreational medications
▶ asthma, epilepsy or diabetes
▶ past surgical operations or serious illnesses.

It is also helpful in cases of trauma or abdominal pain to establish when the patient last ate or drank. This could be relevant for patients who may need a general anaesthetic in the near future.

Observations required for a patient in A&E

As you gain experience you will realise why certain observations are carried out on specific client groups. The table on page 33 shows the presenting conditions and the observations that should be taken.

In addition to the observations listed in the table, it is essential to observe the following points:

1. A BM test for capillary blood sugar should be carried out:

   (a) All diabetic patients as well as all patients presenting with repeated episodes of local skin infections or abscesses

   (b) All patients with a reduced level of consciousness.

2. A peak expiratory flow should be taken on all patients with suspected respiratory disease.

3. Before an ECG is recorded it is important to establish that an appropriate practitioner is available to interpret it, even if the machine has an in-built interpretation facility. An ECG would normally be required on patients who have experienced chest pain

PROBLEM	PULSE	BP	RESPS	BM	PUPILS	TEMP
?CVA/TIA	*	*	*	*	*	*
Abdominal pain	*	*	*	*	*	*
Asthma	*	*	*	*	*	*
Back pain	*	*	*			*
Bleeding tooth socket	*	*	*			*
Burns/scalds > 10%	*	*	*	*		*
Chest pain	*	*	*	*	*	*
Collapse	*	*	*	*	*	*
Compound fractures	*	*	*			*
Diabetic collapse	*	*	*	*	*	*
Difficulty breathing	*	*	*			*
Dislocations	*	*	*			
Earache	*					*
Electric shock	*	*	*	*	*	*
Eye pain/lacrimation	*	*	*		*	*
Facial injury	*	*			*	
Haematuria	*	*	*			*
Haemoptesis	*	*	*			*
Haemotemesis	*	*	*			*
Head injury	*	*	*		*	*
Hip injuries	*	*	*		*	*
Illness	*	*	*	*	*	*
Loin pain	*	*	*			*
Lower limb injuries						
Malaena	*	*	*			*
Minor RTAs	*	*	*		*	
Multiple injuries	*	*	*	*	*	*
Neck injuries	*	*	*			
Overdose	*	*	*	*	*	*
Palpitations	*	*	*	*	*	*
Panic attacks	*	*	*	*	*	*
Psychiatric disorder	*	*	*	*	*	*
Pyrexia	*	*	*	*	*	*
Rash? – cause	*	*	*			*
Simple lacerations						
Sinus problems						*
Unconscious patients	*	*	*	*	*	*
PV bleeding	*	*	*			*

Table 1

where a cardiac cause is suspected or for patients who have collapsed without obvious cause. Some departments delegate ECG recording to specific technicians.

Neurological observations

Neurological observations are used to determine the patient's status relevant to their level of consciousness and responsiveness in association with their pulse, blood pressure and respiratory rate.

This is different to documenting the temperature, pulse and respiration in isolation on a TPR chart. All patients who have an injury or illness that threatens to reduce their level of consciousness should have neurological observations performed.

Those who are or have been unconscious should have serial (repeated) observations performed. In this way, progress against the initial set of observations can be measured.

How to measure neurological observations
Some debate exists around the scoring system used to calculate a Glasgow coma score. Some departments will give a maximum possible score of 14, and others will give 15. This is because those who advocate a score of 15 use an additional sign in the section of 'best motor response' in the form of 'withdrawal' from pain.

Check the scoring system
It is essential that you check whether your department gives a maximum score of 14 or 15. Scoring a patient at a full score of 14 could give the impression that there was something wrong with the patient's level of consciousness, if the department actually used 15 as a maximum score.

Producing a Glasgow coma score
Choose one statement in each section in Table 2 that reflects the patient's response. Allocate the score that goes with it. Add the scores from the three sections to arrive at a total score.

When the scores from each section are added together they will give a Glasgow coma score. A fully conscious patient should achieve a maximum score. Anything lower should be referred to a more senior nurse or doctor for verification.

You will see from the scoring system that the maximum score possible is 15 (or 14 if withdrawal is omitted). The lowest score possible is 3.

eyes open	spontaneously	4
	to speech	3
	to pain	2
	none	1
best verbal response	orientated	5
	confused	4
	odd few words	3
	incomprehensible sounds	2
	none	1
best motor response	obeys commands	6
	localises	5
	withdraws from pain	4
	flexes	3
	extends	2
	none	1
	Total	15

Table 2

It is important to measure the score working through the system in the order listed above, so that the score is not distorted by motor stimulation which may create the false impression of a higher score than is clinically demonstrated.

Children
For children under 10 years old there is a slight variation in measuring the best verbal response by using the following categories:

Orientated	= 5
Unconnected words	= 4
Vocal sounds	= 3
Cries	= 2
None	= 1

Measurement of pupil size and reaction to light
To master this technique properly takes practice and you should never hesitate to seek senior help if you are unsure of what you are looking at.

The first thing is to ensure that you have a good light source, such as a well functioning pen torch.

Prior to shining any light source towards the patient take a couple of moments to have the patient stare at you. In that time you should be able to estimate whether or not both pupils are equal in size. A chart of pupil sizes from 1 mm to 6 mm appears at the left hand side of each Glasgow coma chart. Compare the size of pupils that you see with those on the chart to arrive at a figure in millimetres that can be documented.

At this point, shine the light source directly at each eye in turn. Note whether or not the pupil gets smaller (constricts). A subjective judgement can be made about the pace at which it constricts that falls into the category of 'brisk', 'sluggish' or 'non-reacting'.

Problems with judging pupils
There are several instances where judging a pupil size and reaction can be problematic and they are:

▶ when the patient has a prosthesis (false eye)
▶ when cataracts cloud the appearance of the pupil
▶ when the patient is fearful of light (photophobia)
▶ when trauma or disease has produced swelling around the eye such that it cannot be opened.

Record the lack of a pupil reaction, or failure to test for a reaction, on the chart. You will need to check how your own department documents such findings.

Blood pressure, pulse and respiratory rate

After these tests have been completed a blood pressure, pulse and respiratory rate should be conducted, and recorded, to complete the chart. The respiratory rate is particularly important in a patient who is in shock due to trauma or illness. In some cases it might also be relevant to add such observations as:

temperature
peak expiratory flow
BM reading
oxygen saturation reading

as appropriate to the case. If oxygen saturation is being measured then document whether or not the patient was receiving supplementary oxygen at the time, and if so, how much. Make a note of the patient's appearance – their pallor and skin texture.

While it is important to use the Glasgow coma scoring system accurately it should be remembered that the subjectivity of any system leaves it open to a certain amount of individual interpretation. Physical handicaps such as poor hearing may hamper a patient's response.

When recording the Glasgow coma score on a document other than the chart provided, it is important to note what you are scoring it out of, in other words 15/15 or 14/14. This will eliminate any doubt should a patient be transferred to an area where a different scoring system is used.

Taking a capillary blood sample for glucose estimation

Whatever system is in use for sampling, it is essential to take the universal precaution of wearing gloves. You should do this before taking any sample from a patient.

Several systems of estimation are in use throughout the UK. These range from plain BM test sticks, through to glucometers of various makes and sizes. Find out which system applies in your department.

Remember these simple steps regardless of what the system is:

▶ Have all the equipment you need to hand.

▶ Always explain to the patient what you are going to do, if the patient is able to hear you. This includes unconscious patients, in whom the last sense to go is that of hearing.

▶ Choose an uninjured site to draw the sample from.

▶ Where possible take the sample from the pulp of the little finger in a non-dominant hand. This will hurt less and generate a better sample size than at other digits. In a baby or young infant it may be necessary to draw the sample from the great toe.

▶ Use lancets specifically designed for drawing capillary blood samples. Open needles are inaccurate and may cause a needle-stick injury to yourself if the patient pulls back suddenly and they can also in rare cases cause sensory nerve damage to the patient's finger.

Recording peak expiratory flow and oxygen saturation

Pulse oxymetry is a method used to measure the capillary oxygen level. It is now accepted as part of baseline observations, where there is a potential reduction in oxygen uptake. Examples include shock and respiratory disease.

It is worth taking a few minutes to become familiar with the model of machine used for pulse oxymetry and to be mindful of potential problems in obtaining a reading. These problems are:

▶ The probe has become detached from the patient.
▶ The battery power is insufficient to generate a reading.
▶ The patient has their digit in flexion thus reducing the signal strength to the probe.
▶ A tourniquet may have been applied for other purposes obstructing signals to the probe.

Peak expiratory flow recordings measure the volume of forced expired air in one breath. Readings are easy to obtain so long as the patient cooperates, and their technique is good. An explanation of the technique, and a demonstration of how to blow into the peak expiratory flow meter, should be given to the patient if they have not provided such a sample before.

The patient should be sat as upright as possible, and hold the meter themselves. After a deep inhalation the patient places their mouth completely around the tube and exhales as sharply and as forcibly as possible. They must be careful not to allow their fingers to obstruct the passage of the plastic indicator in models of such type.

A total of three readings are taken consecutively, and the highest is recorded. The technique, whether good or bad, should be documented. The reading is measured in litres per minute. A chart or disc stating the normal expected range of peak expiratory flow readings based on height and weight should be available within your department.

Recording blood pressure, pulse and respiratory rates

Technology for the recording of pulse and blood pressure is available in the departments. However, the advantages of performing an initial set of manually recorded observations are:

▶ The rhythm and volume of the pulse can be detected.
▶ The temperature and texture of the skin can be felt more accurately while the pulse is being recorded.
▶ Abnormal sounds on blood pressure measurement can be heard.
▶ Machine inaccuracies can be identified.

Temperature recording

Temperature recording is most accurately achieved by using a good quality tympanic thermometer.

A tympanic thermometer that elicits an accurate temperature from the ear in just a few seconds is by far the preferred option.

Measuring capillary refill

This is a useful indicator of shock. It is demonstrated through the number of seconds taken for the blood supply to re-enter the end of a finger (distal phalanx), after it has been obstructed for 5 seconds. A refill time greater than 2 seconds should give cause for concern.

To measure capillary refill elevate the patient's hand to a level higher than the heart. Then firmly squeeze the distal phalanx between the end of your thumb and index fingers, being careful to avoid digging your nails into the patient.

Lower the arm to heart level and release the pressure. Note how long it takes for the end of the finger to return to the well perfused colour that was there at the start. Capillary refill measurement is also essential for any sick child. In babies it may be more desirable to measure the capillary refill using the great toe.

Normal values in adult observations

Interpreting recorded observations needs to be done in the context of patient history, and of the basic findings such as that of appearance – as well as on the numerical value of the observations themselves.

For example, a patient may generate normal values of blood pressure and pulse, and yet show a pale pallor and very sweaty skin texture. In such a case, it would be wise to treat the basic visual observations as significant, rather than accept the apparently normal numerical readings. The patient may be compensating for shock.

Table of normal values

The following table gives a range of normal values for a blood pressure, pulse and respiratory rate in an adult:

Blood pressure	100 / 60mmHg – 140 / 90mmHg
BM reading	4mmols – 7mmols
Capillary refill	< 2 seconds
Oxygen saturation	96% – 100% on air
Pulse	60bpm – 100bpm
Respiratory rate	12 – 18 breaths per minute
Temperature	35degrees C – 37degrees C

Summary

▶ Relevant history from numerous sources should be gathered swiftly and accurately.

▶ Baseline observations need to be taken with care and reported to the appropriate personnel.

▶ Always view the patient in the context of history and visual appearance, not just through numerical observations.

▶ Complete your documentation of history and observations accurately, and at the time. Use the format of your own department.

Helping you learn

Progress questions
1. What would be the maximum score that you would calculate for a patient when using the Glasgow coma score?

2. At what temperature would you classify a patient as being hypothermic?

3. How would you obtain a peak flow reading from a patient?

Seminar discussion
How would you deal with a confused patient who refuses to let you record a set of baseline observations?

Practical assignment
Using the equipment available in the department, practise taking a full set of baseline observations on a willing colleague. Do not include a BM reading.

4

Upper Limb Soft Tissue Injuries

One-minute summary – Have a good basic anatomy book handy when reading this chapter. Soft tissue injuries include contusions (bruising), sprains and strains, subluxation and dislocations. Keeping an accurate history, noting the velocity and direction of force, will increase the chances of accurate diagnosis. Damage to underlying structures should always be considered to ensure that an apparently minor injury does not develop into a major injury. Effective pain relief is important, as well as providing basic nursing measures such as elevation, splinting and good wound management. Colour, sensation and the quality of the pulses distal to the site of injury should be assessed.

In this chapter you will learn about:

▶ descriptive terminology in soft tissue injury
▶ frequent soft tissue injuries.

Descriptive terminology

A soft tissue injury is one that causes damage to structures other than bone. These structures include skin, muscle, ligaments, and more seriously, tendons, nerves and joints.

Structures in soft tissues
Before looking at specific injuries it is important to be clear about what the various structures within soft tissues do and what they are made of:

ligament	tough fibrous tissue that holds bones together at joints
tendon	tough fibrous tissue connecting muscle to bone
muscle	tissue made up of fibres that produce contraction for movement
cartilage	tough connective tissue between bones.

The focus of care
After taking an accurate history the main focus of care involves:

41

▶ recognising the need for effective pain relief

▶ assessing the colour, sensation and degree of movement at the site of injury

▶ removal of any mechanical blocks to the circulation, such as rings, bracelets etc.

▶ establishing the presence of distal pulses

▶ immobilising the affected limb and covering open wounds before definitive care.

Signs and symptoms of a soft tissue injury

▶ a history of direct or indirect force

▶ an initial period of pain and immobility

▶ the quick return of at least partial movement at the site of injury

▶ local redness, swelling and pain without deformity of the bone.

An indication of severity in soft tissue injury is when a patient gives a history of hearing a 'crack' at the time of injury, and when they have immediately stopped the activity that they were doing. An example would be coming off the football field without trying to continue the game.

Difficulty of diagnosis

It is often very difficult to arrive at a specific diagnosis immediately. This is because the area of injury can involve many structures that cannot be accurately examined individually until much of the initial pain and swelling has settled to a specific local area.

For this reason quite a few patients return to A&E or to the GP with unresolved symptoms, sometimes weeks and even months after injury. At that later time, a more accurate diagnosis may be made.

In Chapter 3 we emphasised the use of anatomical references when describing landmarks and areas of the body. We can use these same references to describe the direction of force that a limb was taken through during the course of an injury. This information will provide useful clues in identifying the anatomical structures that may be damaged. These are:

In finger and wrist injuries

Hyperflexion   – Direction of force is downwards towards the palm.
Hyperextension – Direction of force is upwards (the wrist bent
                 backwards).

Soft tissue injuries around joints present particular problems. If the integrity of a joint is disrupted then it becomes unstable and thus its ability to function as an effective support for the skeleton is compromised.

When a joint is traumatised several physiological changes can occur which make assessment and diagnosis difficult.

▶ Capillary bleeding can fill the joint space with blood (haemo-arthrosis).

▶ If the joint is encapsulated the capsule can be disrupted.

▶ Synovial and serous fluid can gather (effusion).

▶ Penetrating injuries can retain foreign bodies in the joint.

At this point it is useful to look at the definition of a 'sprain' and a 'strain' because these often cause confusion.

sprain	an injury due to tearing of ligaments at a joint
strain	an injury to muscle or tendon.

Frequent soft tissue injuries

Let's look now at some specific soft tissue injuries that are often found in A&E. We will relate the symptoms and physiology described above to the practical management of these injuries.

Shoulder injuries

The bony frame of the shoulder girdle comprises the scapula, the clavicle and the humerus which in turn are connected through the shoulder joint which is a synovial ball and socket joint capable of abduction, adduction, flexion, extension and rotation. The major groups of soft tissues are:

▶ acromio-clavicular (AC) joint lying just above the shoulder

▶ the rotator cuff comprising of muscles originating from the scapula

▶ the biceps which form the muscular attachment with the humerus

▶ the supraspinatus tendon.

AC joint disruption
This is where the soft tissues in the AC joint above the shoulder have become injured. There are three grades of disruption. Grades two and three require specialist input from an orthopaedic perspective. Diagnosis is usually made initially by clinical findings on examination, and clarified later by radiology using X-ray films. It is unlikely that a junior nurse would be able make such a diagnosis given that X-rays need to be taken as the patient bears weight through the shoulder in order to confirm the grade of injury.

Rotator cuff injury
This is an injury to the group of three muscles that originate from the scapula and form an aponeurosis over the shoulder joint. The supraspinatus and deltoid muscles allow abduction at the shoulder joint; this movement is only partially achievable in rotator cuff injuries, especially where abduction is less than 15°.

Treatment in A&E means applying a broad arm sling and administering appropriate analgesia, pending physiotherapy and further specialist review.

Supraspinatus tendonitis
This is sometimes known as 'painful arc' syndrome. The shoulder is painful on abduction, but more so at night. The condition is caused by repetitive movement rather than by direct injury. It is really more of an inflammatory response than an acute injury from trauma. Treatment in A&E is with a broad arm sling and appropriate analgesia. Intra-articular steroid injections are sometimes required for this condition.

Dislocated shoulder
This is a very painful condition. The shoulder joint has been subjected to indirect trauma resulting in the joint moving out of its anatomical socket. Movement is usually anterior, but a posterior or lateral dislocation can also occur.

Patients present with the good arm supporting the injured side and obvious pain at rest. This is made worse by any attempt to move the injured joint. It is important to provide a trolley or couch for the patient immediately.

Let the patient find a position that is most tolerable. Some patients may find it comfortable to lie prone, with the injured shoulder at the edge of the trolley so that the arm hangs down to produce a natural traction. However, some will not and it is best to allow the patient to find his or her most tolerable position.

It is important to secure early pain relief. This would normally consist of an intravenous opiate accompanied by an anti emetic in adults. Entonox may be helpful while analgesia is being organised followed by X-ray, for which a nurse escort may be required.

Reducing the dislocation

The dislocation must be reduced urgently, because of potential pressure and damage to the nerves and blood vessels that form the brachial plexus which originate in the axilla.

Reduction should be carried out in a location with good resuscitation facilities. This is because respiratory depression could occur as a result of the drugs administered to achieve the reduction

Prior to the reduction beginning, the patient should be placed on high flow oxygen via a non-rebreathing mask. Pulse oxymetry and cardiac monitoring should be established. Loose dentures and spectacles should be removed and a secure canula should be flushed prior to administering any drugs.

Elbow injuries

As a hinge joint the elbow provides movement between the lower end of the humerus and the ulna. It also:

▶ is a ball and socket. This provides articulation between the lower end of the humerus and the inferior radio-ulna joint at the wrist, allowing the movements of **pronation** and **supination**.

▶ is capable at the elbow joint itself only of movement in flexion and extension.

▶ has an **olecranon** process at the posterior end of the ulna protected by a sack (**bursar**).

▶ accommodates soft tissues. These include the insertions of the triceps muscles, the brachial artery and vein and the point at which sensation through the **ulna nerve** can be accessed, commonly known as the 'funny' bone.

Joint effusion

This is a condition where fluid gathers in the elbow joint following trauma. The fluid can consist of blood or serous fluid, and is recognisable by a soft mobile swelling at the joint, which is painful to the touch.

Treatment depends upon first excluding any fracture. We must then balance the relief that aspirating the fluid might bring, against the potential risk of infection when a puncture wound is created during the aspiration procedure.

Although effusions will eventually reabsorb if left without aspiration, it is often painful. It can also be dangerous, in view of vascular occlusion, to treat all such conditions conservatively.

Olecranon bursitis

This is a condition where the normally even bursar – the sac, which covers the olecranon – distends into a bulbous like deformity. This is due to the distension caused by excessive synovial fluid secretion.

The condition results from pressure on the olecranon, either in acute trauma or in long term repeated situations, where for example a student has leaned on a desk for long periods. Occasionally it is also caused by infection.

Treatment is normally conservative. At most it involves a broad arm sling for 24 to 48 hours for the purpose of rest, followed by gentle mobilisation. A surgical repair is rare and would not be a first line A&E treatment.

Olecranon bursitis resulting from infection is managed with the appropriate antibiotics. These may be given intravenously in more serious cases. Patients with olecranon bursitis should have a temperature recorded to confirm or exclude an infective cause.

Tennis elbow

When an object is gripped, the extensor tendons of the wrist are used and their origin is in the lateral epicondyle. Repeated use gives rise to a partial tear of the fibres at the epicondyle. This results in pain on the lateral side of the elbow, which is often dull and aching in nature. Direct pressure on the elbow is painful but X-rays usually show nothing abnormal. First line treatment in A&E is based on rest and anti-inflammatory analgesics.

Some patients find a broad arm sling less helpful than others in this condition.

Wrist injuries

The wrist joint is a complex one. It begins at the distal end of the radius and ulna, and comprises:

(a) eight carpal bones

(b) five metacarpal bones that span the body of the hand.

(c) an interosseous membrane that is a tough fibrous membrane running through the forearm between the radius and ulna

(d) the extensor retinaculum which forms a fibrous belt across the wrist joint under which tendons and other structures pass

(e) medial and lateral ligaments

(f) extensor and flexor tendons

(g) vascular supply from the radial and ulna arteries and veins

(h) a nerve supply from the radial, ulna and median nerves.

Hyperextension or hyperflexion in the wrist
Among soft tissue injuries resulting from trauma, most of the presentations to A&E offer a history of hyperextension or hyperflexion from a fall or trauma through rotational force.

Soft tissue injuries in the wrist joint are largely diagnosed through a process of exclusion. Assessment seeks to exclude:

1. the presence of a bony injury (fracture)

2. a dislocation of the lunate which is a rare but devastating injury to miss

3. rupture of the medial or lateral ligaments that would threaten the stability of the wrist joint

4. neurovascular compromise.

Scaphoid injury
The scaphoid bone is the largest of the eight carpal bones. Its blood supply comes from a branch of the radial artery. The bone is shaped like a boat, and when a fracture occurs it is normally sustained through the waist of the scaphoid.

A fracture is therefore problematic, because the blood supply can be compromised if the blood to flow to the scaphoid is impeded.

Unfortunately the appearance of a fracture on X-ray may not be apparent for up to 14 days. This can give the wrong initial impression, that there is simply a soft tissue injury. Any patient who gives a history of trauma associated with scaphoid tenderness is normally treated with a period of immobilisation, either in a support bandage, splint or plaster. A repeat X-ray is obtained within two weeks after injury, when any fracture will show itself radiologically.

Tenosinovitis

This is an inflammatory condition of the extensor tendons. It results from repetitive movement of the wrist, usually over a substantial period of time. Pain tends to be focused on the dorsum of the wrist and forearm on the radial side nearest the thumb. The area can often be hot to the touch.

In more severe cases it may be possible to hear crepitus on extension at the wrist joint. Initial treatment is to provide support for the wrist. This is normally done with a support bandage or a futuro splint. In extreme cases a plaster of Paris cast may be used, together with non steroidal anti inflammatory drugs such as Ibuprofen or Naproxen. In severe cases a local steroid injection may be indicated.

The hand

Gross anatomy of the hand

In terms of gross anatomy the hand consists of:

▶ five long bones known as metacarpals that extend from the carpal bones in the wrist down to their distal end

▶ five metocarpophalangeal joints

▶ five digits which are known as the thumb, index, middle, ring and little fingers

▶ a proximal and a distal interphalangeal joint in each finger

▶ an interphalangeal joint in each thumb

▶ a proximal, middle and distal phalanx in each finger and a proximal and distal phalanx at each thumb

▶ a nail emerging from a nail bed at each digit.

Soft tissues of the hand

In terms of soft tissues the hand consists of:

1. a labyrinth of extensor and flexor tendons

2. sensory and motor nerves

3. arterial and venous blood vessels

4. ligaments supporting the joints which are themselves surrounded by a joint capsule

5. an area of cartilage running through the volar aspect of the digits known as the volar plate.

Hand injuries can be devastating to patients who suddenly find themselves incapable of earning a living, or carrying out essential life tasks at home. It cannot be emphasised enough how important it is to have any hand injury properly assessed by an experienced nurse or doctor, before discharging a soft tissue injury home.

The usual cause of soft tissue injury to the hand is a direct blow, crush injury, or hyperextension or hyperflexion at a joint.

Sprains and strains
Hyperflexion and hyperextension are the usual form of these injuries. They produce local swelling and pain and restricted movement due to pain at the joint affected, and often in the immediate surrounding joints.

So long as the sensation and blood supply to the hand distal to the site of injury is adequate, most of these uncomplicated injuries settle with just symptomatic treatment. This normally takes the form of a support bandage and a high arm sling for a day or so. These promote the venous drainage that will help to reduce swelling.

It is also important to advise the patient to take simple analgesia as required and that the hand be moved again quite quickly. This should avoid complications of stiffness at the joints after the initial injury has healed.

Ligament injuries
Lateral and medial ligaments surround the joints within the hand and through the joints of the digits. Damage is usually due to excessive mechanisms of hyperextension. An example would be when a football is saved when it is kicked at speed towards the outstretched hand.

The radio-collateral and ulna-collateral ligaments at the base of the thumb are particularly problematic. This is because they are important in enabling us to grip, and also because of the surgical repair needed in case of rupture.

A ligament injury at this site that if left uncorrected for a week or more generates major difficulties in the process of surgical repair.

Mallet finger

This is a rupture of the extensor tendons at the level of the distal phalanx. It can occur in any finger, but is most commonly found at the index and middle fingers. It does not require significant force to produce this injury and some patients present following such gentle trauma as fastening a button.

The injury is diagnosed by clinical examination alone. It will be obvious that the distal phalanx is in flexion and will not extend, despite the patient's best efforts. Extension at all other joints is normal in mallet finger deformity. Treatment involves correctly applying a mallet splint to maintain a position of slight extension of the distal phalanx. This should be retained for a period of six weeks, at which a review takes place.

The patient should not remove the splint at all during the six weeks. Prognosis is generally poor in this injury. Surgical repair at this level is difficult, and rarely indicated.

Subungual haematoma

This is where a clot of blood forms under a nail following direct trauma. For example the patient may have hit the digit with a hammer during DIY or crushed the finger when closing a door.

These injuries are painful due to the pressure exerted by the collection of blood. The treatment is to **trephine** the nail. This involves burning a hole through the nail in order to release the blood.

This brings about instant relief for the patient who is often very apprehensive of this treatment. If an underlying fracture is suspected or confirmed, then antibiotics should be supplied. This is because the hole that has been produced technically makes the fracture compound.

Caution is required by the nurse during trephining because the release of blood under pressure can produce a forceful spillage and **goggles should be worn by the nurse as a precaution.**

Summary

▶ The movements at the joints within the upper limb will depend upon the type of joint it is.

▶ History is important in establishing the type of force and direction of the injury.

▶ Crush injuries can endanger the blood supply distal to the area of injury, and should be dealt with by senior staff.

Helping you learn

Progress questions

1. What movements are possible at the elbow joint and why?

2. Name the eight carpal bones.

3. Why is an injury to the base of the thumb significant?

Seminar discussion

How would you determine the range of movement in the finger of a patient with learning difficulties?

Practical assignment

With the help of a colleague, take all of the joints in the upper limb through their natural range of movement, and state the term for the movement you produce.

Lower Limb Soft Tissue Injuries

One-minute summary – Extending from the hips to the toes the lower limbs provide the facility to bear the weight of the body in standing and walking. Sprains, strains, dislocations and neurovascular injury can arise in the same way as for the upper limbs except that the degree of immobility for the patient can be increased. Nursing care is focused on achieving a safe and comfortable position for the patient on arrival, early appropriate pain relief in lieu of an accurate diagnosis, and appropriate treatment, including any necessary referral or follow up. The healing time for a soft tissue injury should not be underestimated. Clear instructions should be given about the principles of rest, ice, compression and elevation during the early days of the healing process. At the time of writing current research challenges the historical merits of compression.

In this chapter you will learn about:

▶ management of hip injuries
▶ management of knee injuries
▶ management of lower leg injuries
▶ management of ankle and foot injuries.

Management of hip injuries

The hip joint sits in the acetabulum, a cavity situated at either side of the pelvis. As a ball and socket joint the hip is capable of movements in flexion, extension, abduction and adduction.

The femur is the long bone extending from the hip joint. Fractures to this area will be discussed in the later chapter on major trauma. Soft tissues in the hip incorporate large muscle groups that include:

▶ the biceps
▶ sartorius
▶ vastas
▶ quadriceps muscles.

On the medial side of the hip lie the femoral vein artery and nerve, with the sciatic nerve running through the length of the femur as it extends distal to it.

Contusions and haematomas

Bruising to the hip is common when trauma occurs, because of the abundance of soft tissues present. As a weight bearing joint, the hip sustains significant trauma in falls and it is usually direct trauma that accounts for most hip injuries. Haematoma formation although painful generally reabsorbs without treatment.

However, it is important to exclude a fracture in any trauma to the hip where a patient fails to bear weight, especially if the patient is frail and elderly. Consideration needs to be given to the possibility of a bony injury to the pelvis where a patient fails to bear weight on an injured hip. This is particularly relevant to frail elderly patients where a fracture of the Pubic Remi can result in pain around the hip.

Irritable hip

This is primarily, but not exclusively, a problem in children. Strictly speaking it is a medical condition rather than a soft tissue injury. However, patients present believing that the symptoms of heat, pain and discomfort on movement must have emanated from an injury, but this is is rarely the case. A temperature should be recorded in these patients.

Dislocated hip

An extremely painful injury where the hip joint has moved anteriorly, posteriorly or laterally from its natural position. Clinical signs include rotation of the foot, usually externally, and intense guarding of the hip by the patient. Pain is increased at any attempt of movement around the joint.

The danger with dislocations at the hip joint is compression or damage to surrounding blood vessels and nerves. This is why it is important to check distal pulses regularly, before reducing the dislocation.

The nursing care for dislocations of the hip includes:

▶ making the patient as comfortable as possible
▶ enabling the patient to self administer Entonox if clincially safe to do so prior to intravenous opiate analgesia and anti emetic.

After an X-ray has confirmed a dislocation, and excluded a fracture, the reduction is carried out as a matter of urgency. This is done under sedation, as for dislocated shoulders, or with a general anaesthetic if sedation does not work.

Management of knee injuries

The knee is a synovial hinge joint capable of flexion and extension. It comprises

1. the distal end of the femur, with a tendon extending through muscle to the patella (a sesamoid bone situated centrally over the knee joint)
2. the cruciate ligaments
3. the medial and lateral collateral ligaments
4. two semilunar cartilage (menisci), one medial and one lateral.

Ligament strain in the knee
Policies around the criteria for X-ray in knee injuries may differ between departments however some may apply the 'Ottawa' rules which broadly advocate X-ray in patients who have sustained trauma to the knee which has resulted in the patient being unable to bear weight for four steps unaided in the department or where there is isolated tenderness over the Patella and head of fibula or an inability to flex the knee to 90 degrees. Patients over the age of 55 are considered to be particularly vulnerable to potential bony injury. Rotational force or direct blows to the knee can produce damage to the ligaments which, as with other joints, will threaten the integrity of the joint. Pain and inability to bear weight are often accompanied by guarding or holding the knee due to the level of pain and fear of further injury.

It is often necessary to place these patients on trolleys rather than wheelchairs. This is to give them adequate support at the knee joint before treatment.

Treatment
Treatment may involve admission under the orthopaedic team, if the joint is clinically unstable when examined, because a surgical repair may be necessary. In lesser cases immobilisation of the knee is achieved

using a range of methods including support bandage, Robert Jones bandage, Richard Splint, or plaster of Paris.

It could be argued that a significant ligament tear in the knee is not a minor injury.

Tear of the meniscus

A torn meniscus will produce pain on extension. This is because, as trauma occurs, synovial fluid is secreted in greater quantities, resulting in swelling at the joint. This in turn impedes the function of the quadriceps muscle, which leads to the patient feeling that the knee is unstable.

If a portion of torn meniscus is lodged inside the joint then clicking and locking of the knee can be felt. If the knee is examined by an experienced nurse or doctor then evidence of clicking can be significant in producing a diagnosis of a menisceal injury.

The surgical removal of the meniscus is the usual treatment; the meniscus has no blood supply of its own for the purpose of healing. Treatment in A&E is the same as for ligament strains, rather than surgery which is accessed via an elective route.

Effusion/haemoarthrosis

The collection of synovial fluid or blood in the joint space as a response to trauma is self limiting. It is evident by comparing the injured knee with the other knee and palpating the area gently to ensure that the swelling is soft. Treatment is the same as for a similar problem at the elbow joint outlined in the previous chapter.

Loose body

Fragments within the knee joint may break off in response to trauma or excessive strain. As a result loose bodies can form anywhere in the joint.

The patient may give a long history of pain on walking, and clicking or locking of the knee. They may say they can usually deal with it themselves until the problem forces them to seek professional help at A&E. In such a case, the presence of a loose body is usually worth considering. An X-ray, Arthroscopy or scan will usually demonstrate the loose body's location and size. Again, the most effective treatment is surgical removal which is usually done as a day case on the waiting list.

Pre-patella bursitis

As with the elbow, the patella is lined with several bursae. Under continuous pressure this will produce an effusion and inflammatory response. It can also have an infective cause in some cases.

Treatment is a little more aggressive than for the elbow because of the weight bearing function required of the knee. Rest elevation, and intravenous antibiotics where appropriate, is the treatment of choice. In cases where the patient is systemically well and swelling does not involve tracking it may be that treatment with oral antibiotics would be considered.

Dislocated patella

This is an injury occurring when the patella is shifted from the central position within the knee to a medial or lateral position in which the ligaments fail to support it. The injury is characterised by pain and immobility as well as a visual deformity at the knee joint. Care is the same as for a dislocated hip. The patient sometimes finds it helpful to have a rolled up blanket placed under the knee joint on arrival.

Management of lower leg injuries

Gastrocnemius tear

Joining from the knee to the ankle, the gastrocnemius muscle in the calf has a lateral and medial head as well as a tendon insertion.

This is an important muscle. Trauma will produce an inability to bear weight due to acute pain. There will be swelling at the back of the calf. The pain often extends the entire length of the calf, increasing around the proximal area near to the knee.

Care must be taken when taking the history to ensure that the calf is not red and hot and that the patient does not have chest pain or shortness of breath, consistent with symptoms of a deep vein thrombosis.

Compartment syndrome

The muscles of the lower leg are divided into four compartments. Compartment syndrome arises from a herniation of one of the muscles through the compartment to cause bleeding and oedema. It results in compression on the structures close to that compartment. Symptoms include a tight swollen 'unyielding' area around the affected compartment, and acute pain aggravated by movement. In extreme cases it may involve neurovascular compromise.

Treatment after a firm diagnosis of compartment syndrome mainly involves surgery. Such patients are referred to an orthopaedic team for further management.

Management of ankle and foot injuries

The ankle joint allows articulation between the tibia and fibula. It involves the seven tarsal bones:

1. the talus
2. calcaneum
3. navicular
4. cuboid
5. medial cuniform
6. intermediate cuniform
7. lateral cuniform.

Soft tissues include the Achilles tendon, the medial and lateral ligaments and the talofibular ligament complex. Nerve supply is from the branches of the tibial nerve, and blood supply from branches of the tibial arteries and veins.

Sprained ankle

Inversion is the most common mechanism for this injury, so common in sport. As the ankle inverts (turns inwards) the ligaments are stretched beyond the point at which they are designed to go.

The result is usually pain and swelling local to the lateral maleolus. This is the point on the distal fibula that is prominent at the distal end.

In isolation this injury will be unlikely to involve bone. However, a bony fragment can be avulsed in severe trauma. Where such an incidence is suspected an X-ray is indicated. As with knee injuries mentioned on page 56 a set of clinical prediction rules (the Ottawa rules) have been produced to suggest a possible criteria for X-ray. These broadly include an inability to bear weight for four steps, tenderness over the posterior aspect of the lateral maleolus or an associated tenderness over the medial maleolus. Treatment for an ankle sprain is based on the principles of rest, ice, compression and elevation (RICE). The patient should be told that the injury will take at least four weeks to heal properly and that some appropriate simple analgesia may be helpful.

The integrity of the ankle joint should be assessed. This should include an assessment of the talofibular ligament complex. Caution is required with patients who complain of tenderness on the medial side and at the back of the ankle, or at the base of the 5th metatarsal, for reasons that are explained below.

Ankle dislocations

These can be posterior, lateral or anterior. They are recognisable by a marked deformity at the ankle joint, coupled with acute pain and immobility. Reduction of this dislocation is urgent owing to the compression of blood vessels and nerves that feed the foot.

It is not uncommon for ankle dislocations to be reduced before an X-ray is taken, because of the urgency. Nursing care is the same as for dislocation of the hip.

Achilles tendon rupture

The Achilles tendon can be palpated at the back of the ankle as it lines the distal end of the tibia posteriorly. Any examination of the ankle should include palpation along the Achilles to ensure that no steps or gaps are present and that the patient is not tender at that point.

Complete rupture of the Achilles is a devastating injury requiring surgical repair. Rupture is usually preceded by a feeling of sharp intense pain at the back of the ankle and the patient describes it as if someone clouted them with a hammer. Weight bearing is not possible in complete Achilles rupture.

The foot

The foot comprises five metatarsals and five digits which are known as the great, 2nd, 3rd, 4th and 5th toes. The gross anatomy of the foot is very much as for the hand, though its function is nowhere near as precise.

5th metatarsal injury

At the proximal end (base) of the 5th metatarsal there is a vulnerability to fracture when the ankle is inverted in injury. It is therefore important to look for bruising or tenderness at the base of the 5th metatarsal before dismissing an ankle sprain as purely soft tissue in origin. Treatment varies according to the degree of swelling. Mild injuries are supported with an appropriate bandage and swollen injuries are supported in plaster of Paris for three to four weeks.

Summary

▶ Soft tissue injuries to lower limbs produce greater immobility for patients than those of the upper limbs.

▶ Dislocations at the hip, knee and ankle are acute emergencies requiring urgent reduction.

▶ When checking for foot pulses, remember to compare both limbs.

▶ Bear in mind the need for good effective analgesia in lower limb soft tissue injuries.

Helping you learn

Progress questions
1. Name two common injuries to the knee.
2. List the names of the tarsal bones.
3. What is the most common cause of irritable hip?

Seminar discussion
Evaluate how much difficulty the presence of chronic arthritis might present when assessing a lower limb injury.

Practical assignment
Ask a willing colleague to act as a patient for you. Pinpoint the landmarks that you would expect to be tender following an inversion injury to the right ankle.

6

Management of Fractures

One-minute summary – A fracture is a break in the continuity of the bone. The clinical signs of a fracture include pain, swelling, redness, deformity and crepitus on movement. The priorities in nursing care are to provide a safe comfortable position for the limb to be immobilised, correct use of immobilisation devices, and early appropriate effective analgesia. Distal pulses and skin colour should always be checked and abnormalities quickly reported. The correct definitive treatment or referral follows escort to X-ray for those who have had opiate analgesia. Baseline systemic observations are important to identify early signs of shock. All open wounds should be covered immediately on arrival.

In this chapter you will learn about:

▶ the terminology of fractures
▶ the principles of treatment
▶ managing specific fractures
▶ how a fracture heals
▶ nursing care in fracture management.

Terminology

closed	not exposed to the atmosphere via a wound.
compound	exposed to the atmosphere via a wound.
undisplaced	the bone remains in line at the fracture site.
displaced	the bone is out of line at the fracture site.
intra articular	the fracture involves a joint.
comminuted	multiple fragments of bone at the fracture site.
incomplete	fracture through one side of the bone leaving the other intact.
greenstick	fractures (incomplete) found in children.

Terminology is also used to describe the pathway that a fracture takes through a bone.

1. transverse   a horizontal line through the bone
2. oblique   fracture at anything other than right angles through a bone
3. spiral   a vertical fracture taking a circular path through a bone
4. impacted   the two bone ends are pushed into each other at the fracture site.

Principles of treatment

These are the principles for dealing with patients who present with suspected fractures.

1. A position of safety where they are unlikely to aggravate the injury further.

2. Observations and assessment for potential major injuries including neurovascular injury.

3. Covering any open wounds.

4. Early effective pain relief.

5. Temporary immobilisation through splinting or positioning prior to X-ray.

6. Obtaining accurate X-ray views of the fracture site and other sites relevant to it.

7. Appropriate definitive management of the fracture.

Fractures that are displaced require manipulation either through closed or open reduction. Compound fractures require surgical debridement.

Managing specific fractures

The policies for the management of fractures will vary according to the facilities available within each hospital, and according to the clinical protocols that have been locally agreed.

The following table relates to the management of fractures within the Leicester Royal Infirmary at the time of writing. Management will vary according to local policy and facilities.

STRUCTURE	INJURY	TYPE	Rx	BEWARE	DISPOSAL
SC Jt.	Dislocation	anterior	BAS		#C
		posterior		mediastinal trauma	Ortho SHO
Clavicle	Fracture	mid 1/3	BAS	severe displacement	#C Ortho SHO Ortho SHO
				? skin viability	
		lateral 1/3	BAS		#C
				displaced	Ortho SHO
AC Jt.	Dislocation	grade 1	BAS		GP PRN
		grade 2	BAS		#C
		grade 3			Ortho SHO
Scapula	Fracture	non articular	BAS		#C
		glenoid		underlying trauma	Ortho SHO
Gleno Humeral Jt.	Dislocation	anterior	MR BAS	axillary nerve	#C
		posterior	MR BAS	axillary nerve	#C
	# Dislocation				Ortho SHO
Humerus	Fracture	tuberosity	BAS		#C
		tuberosity, displaced			Ortho SHO
		neck	C&C		#C
		shaft	U Slab, C&C	radial nerve	#C
Elbow	Supracondylar	undisplaced	AEP	neurovascular	#C
Femur	NOF				NOF SHO
	Shaft		Splint and block		Ortho SHO
Knee	Haemarthrosis				Ortho SHO
	Effusion				A&E Clinic 10/7
	Ligament injury				Ortho SHO

STRUCTURE	INJURY	TYPE	Rx	BEWARE	DISPOSAL
Patella	Dislocation	acute	MR Cylinder POP		#C
		recurrent	Tibigrip		#C
	Fracture	intact exensor	POP BS		#C
		disrupted extensor			Ortho SHO
Tibia	Shaft			compartment	Ortho SHO
Fibula	Shaft		BKBS	diastastis	#C
Ankle	Lat Maleolus #	undisplaced	BKBS	displacement	#C
	Bi Maleolar	undisplaced	BKBS	displacement	#C
	Either	displaced			Ortho SHO
Talus	Fracture	undisplaced	BKBS NWB		#C
		displaced			Ortho SHO
Calcaneum	Fracture			swelling	Ortho SHO
Other Tarsal bones	Fracture		BKWP		#C
	Dislocation			lisfranc	Ortho SHO
Metatarsal	Fracture		BKWP	swelling	#C
	# Styloid		Tibigrip		#C
Phalanges	Extra articular		Symptomatic		Discharge
	Intra articular		Symptomatic		#C
		displaced			Ortho SHO
	Articular #	undisplaced	C&C		#C
		displaced			Ortho SHO
	Dislocation		MR BAS		#C
	Olecranon	displaced			Ortho SHO
		undisplaced			#C

STRUCTURE	INJURY	TYPE	Rx	BEWARE	DISPOSAL
Radius and Ulnar	Radial head	undisplaced	C&C		#C
	Radial neck	<30' angle	C&C		#C
		>30' angle			Ortho SHO
	Radial shaft	undisplaced	AEP		#C
		displaced		Galeazzi	Ortho SHO
	Ulnar shaft	undisplaced	AEP		#C
		fisplaced		Monteggia	Ortho SHO
	Colles	undisplaced	BS		#C
		displaced			Ortho SHO
		greenstick	BS		#C
		buckle	Symptomatic		#C
	Smiths				Otho SHO
	Either styloid	undisplaced	BS		#C
Carpus	Scaphoid	fractured	Colles BS		#C
		suspected	Tibigrip		A+E Clinic 10/7
	Other Carpal	fractured	BS		#C
Metacarpals	Thumb	extra articula	Scaphoid POP		#C
		Bennett's			Ortho SHO
	NECKS				
	Index/Middle	<20' flex	Neigbour Strap	Rotation	#C
		>20' Flex	MR	Rotation	#C
	Ring/Little	<70' flex	Neigbour Strap	Rotation	#C
		>70' flex	MR	Rotation	#C
	SHAFTS		Volar POP	Rotation	#C
Phalanges	Shafts	displaced	MR + splint		A+E Clinic 1/52
		undisplaced	Splint		A+E Clinic 1/52
	Mallet		Mallet splint		A+E Clinic 3/52
Pelvis	# Rami Only		Analgesia		GP FU
	ANY Other #		Pos Ex Fix	BLOOD LOSS	Ortho SHO
Hip	Dislocation	traumatic		Sig trauma	Ortho SHO
		post THR			Ortho SHO

NB. # -VE Hip pain that needs admission is arranged by Ortho SHO.

Less common fractures

There are some other fractures that are less commonly seen but still worth mentioning for more advanced learning. They are:

Galeazzi fracture   Fracture to the shaft of the radius with dislocation of the inferior radio-ulna joint.

Monteggia fracture Fracture of the ulna with dislocation at the head of the radius.

How a fracture heals

► Bleeding at the site produces a haematoma.

► A fibrous framework of blood vessels forms in the haematoma.

► From this begins the formation of osteoid tissue due to the deposits of calcium.

► Ossification rebuilds the bone (osteoblasts) producing a calus formation.

► Osteoclasts remove unwanted material as remodelling occurs.

Nursing care

In this section we will look at the key aspects of nursing care in fracture management.

Pain relief

Patients who sustain fractures are almost always in pain. It is important to deliver the correct analgesia quickly and accurately. Analgesia in children is covered in the chapter on paediatrics.

In adults there are several options that can be considered. Much will depend upon the degree to which the patient perceives pain as to what drug is used and in what dosage. Pain is an individual experience and there is no objective tool to measure it. One way of understanding an individual patient's pain is to create a 'pain scale'. This seeks to put a score of 10 on the worst pain that the patient has ever had in his life and zero on no pain at all, hence establishing a comparative score for the pain of the fracture.

Undisplaced fractures of the fingers and toes that do not involve dislocation may well respond to oral analgesia such as Co-Codamol. This can also be taken in conjunction with an anti inflammatory drug such as Naproxen or Ibuprofen. Other mild to moderate oral analgesics include Dihydrocodene or even simple Paracetamol.

It is worth remembering that non steroidal anti-inflammatory drugs such as Naproxen or Ibuprofen are not recommended in asthmatics, or for patients with peptic ulceration.

Displaced fractures and fractures above the level of the digits often require intravenous analgesia. This is administered through a secure cannula that is sited in a large peripheral vein. Intramuscular analgesia should be avoided in A&E. It is slow to absorb and often ineffective in the initial stages of care. This makes further doses necessary that can result in accumulative doses several hours down the line.

Morphine is the drug of choice for pain relief in severe bony pain.

Preparation for drugs

Intravenous morphine should always be drawn up to a solution of 10mls. This way a titrated dose can be given incrementally in line with the patient's response. For example, a solution of morphine, which came from pharmacy as 10mg per ml, should have 9mls of normal saline or water for injection added to it to make a 10ml solution.

The administration of an anti emetic such as Metochlopramide (Maxalon) is mandatory with any initial dose of opiates in adults. The syringes containing the drugs should all be labelled stating the number of mg per ml before checking and administration.

If a patient is to receive intravenous opiates then a set of baseline observations should be taken. These should include a respiratory rate because opiates depress the respiratory function and a baseline is needed for comparison.

For the same reason any patient who looks unwell or is unduly pale in colour before or after analgesia should be given supplementary oxygen. The patient should be observed carefully, and a nurse escort provided to X-ray, fracture clinic or to the ward if admission is indicated.

Splints

The amount of splinting that a fracture site requires in A&E depends upon the following factors:

1. how much exposure to medical examinations the site will have over the initial period in A&E

2. how much movement it would be safe to allow while the patient is taken through the system

3. how the circulation of blood can best be preserved, or haemorrhage best controlled

4. how long it is likely to be before definitive care can be provided

5. in what position the patient is most comfortable.

Types of splint
There are many splints on the market for use in fracture management. Some of the best known are:

Bradford sling	used to elevate the hand and the upper limb
air splint	transparent compressible splints for upper and lower limbs
box splint	a wooden splint joined by a bandage tie around the affected limb
Loxley splint	a soft plastic splint version of the box splint
Sager splint	an adjustable metal splint for immobilising femoral shaft fractures
Thomas splint	a metal splint with a padded circular ring for femoral shaft fractures
hare splint	an adapted version of the Thomas splint
plaster of Paris	either as a temporary back slab or permanent treatment for the fracture.

Application of splints
The application of a splint is a skill that comes through careful observation and clinical experience. However, the following tips might be helpful.

▶ Explain and reassure the patient before applying a splint.

▶ Entonox should be self administered by the patient if systemic pain relief has not been given, or if temporary additional analgesia is needed during splinting.

▶ Avoid moving areas that have bone protruding near to the surface or through the skin. This is to avoid making a closed fracture open (compound).

▶ Never have the patient support the weight of a fractured limb. Always have a colleague support it with you.

▶ Ensure that you can easily reach the distal pulses without lengthy investments of time in splint removal.

The Thomas splint

Of all the splints described above, the Thomas splint is often the hardest to apply. It takes time to measure the size required, and to assemble the various components that come with it. The method for application is detailed below, to help you when you assemble and apply your first splint under the supervision of a more experienced nurse.

In order to assemble and apply a Thomas splint you will need:

1. one tape measure
2. one adult or child skin traction kit with bandage included
3. three Velcro slings
4. one appropriately sized Thomas splint
5. traction cord to tie the splint
6. two wooden spatulas
7. one or two pillows.

Step by step:

▶ Measure the uninjured leg from the head of the femur to the end of the calcaneum on the uninjured side and add 3 inches.

▶ Measure the circumference of the uninjured thigh around the widest point and add 2 inches.

▶ Select a right or left leg splint as appropriate that matches closely as possible the measurements taken.

▶ Fold the Velcro slings through the splint at three points, leaving a gap at the level of the knee. Use the traction cord to secure the slings.

▶ With care, and appropriate analgesia, gently straighten the injured leg out as far as possible. Have a colleague maintain traction. You may wish to maintain traction first time round to observe the application.

▶ Shave any excessive hairs on the sides of the injured leg and apply the skin traction cutting a V shape on the upper and lower ends at the level of the knee.

► Apply the bandage from thigh to ankle, leaving a gap at the knee.

► Maintain traction while gently lifting the leg to slide the splint into place.

► Tie the skin traction cord to the end of the splint by crossing it over, and alternately under, the side frames of the splint.

► Place a spatula in the distal knot of the traction cord. Rotate to tighten it, leaving the spatula secured across the frame of the splint.

► Place some padding under the knee for comfort and to prevent sores.

► Raise the patient's leg onto one or two pillows.

Compound fractures
Compound fractures require antibiotics and these are usually administered intravenously as an initial dose followed by oral medication later. The usual drugs of choice are Cefuroxime 750mg – 1500mg and Metronidazole 500mg by 100ml infusion.

Plaster of Paris
The use of plaster of Paris in fracture immobilisation is a skill requiring manual dexterity that only comes with experience. We cannot describe the method of applying each individual type of plaster in this book, but from the list below you can work out what you would like to learn from experienced staff who plaster on a regular basis.

Back slabs and full plasters
    Colles
    below elbow
    above elbow
    U-slab
    volar slab
    above knee
    below knee.

More advanced plasters
    scaphoid (less used now than in the past)
    cylinder plasters
    aquinas plasters.

Plasters can also be 'moulded', usually by medical staff who require firm support for a manipulated or potentially mobile fracture. It is also possible to split or bi-valve a plaster as a compromise between a back slab and a full plaster in some long bone fractures.

Patients who require surgical management of their fractures may either go straight to theatre from A&E or go first to an orthopaedic ward prior to surgery. In either case you should ask the orthopaedic team whether the patient is able to eat or drink – due to anaesthetics in the future. Additional injectable analgesia may be required for patients who need to remain 'nil by mouth'. Also, dextrose infusions may be needed for diabetic patients who are unable to eat or drink.

Summary

▶ A fracture is a break in the continuity of a bone. Within this definition there are several types of fracture, including open or closed, undisplaced or displaced.

▶ The direction of force determines the pattern the fracture will take through the bone, for example transverse or spiral.

▶ Initial early effective immobilisation and pain relief is imperative.

▶ It is important to assess systemic and neurovascular compromise at all stages of management in A&E.

▶ Fractures follow a specific physiological process in healing.

Helping you learn

Progress questions

1. Describe three directions that a fracture can take through a bone.

2. How would you prepare an injection of morphine for intravenous administration to a patient?

3. How would you measure a patient for a Thomas splint to the right leg?

Seminar discussions

1. How would you deal with a patient who was clearly in pain but who refused any offer of analgesia?

2. What implications are there for a patient who has sustained a fracture and therefore needs analgesia but who has consumed a large volume of alcohol?

Practical assignments

1. Find an experienced colleague and assemble a Thomas splint ready for application.

2. Identify all the palpable distal pulses on yourself. Try to assess your own capillary refill.

Wound Care In A&E

One-minute summary – There are eight classifications of wound that require specific management. All wounds need assessment to check for trauma to underlying structures, and for systemic problems arising from blood loss, rupture or foreign body retention. All wounds should be covered in A&E, except when clinical treatment is in progress. Any treatments should be carried out in conditions of asepsis, as far as possible. Treatments for wounds include dressings, wound tissue adhesives, steristrip closures, sutures and staples. Wounds heal by first intention or granulation. Factors that delay healing include the general health of the patient, the acquisition of infection and the effectiveness of wound closure.

In this chapter you will learn:

▶ the classification of wounds
▶ the assessment of wounds
▶ types of wound closure
▶ practical methods of wound closure.

Classification of wounds

Definition
A wound is a break in the continuity of the skin.

Classification
There are eight classifications of wounds:

Contusion	A bruise.
Abrasion	A wound caused by friction that results in the removal of or damage to the epidermis.
Laceration	Occurs through the epidermis and dermis of the skin. Laceration can be incisional, irregular, or a flap wound.

Puncture	A small circular point of entry through the skin.
Burn	Damage to layers of the skin caused by dry heat.
Scald	Damage to layers of the skin caused by wet heat.
Gunshot	A penetrating wound caused by a firearm.
Degloving	Underlying structures are exposed following the complete and often intact removal of the skin when the limb is withdrawn from a crush between two surfaces.

Wound assessment

After taking a history, there follows the process of wound assessment. This includes visual inspection, the possibility of X-rays, covering the wound, and elevating any heavily bleeding limb.

Visual inspection
The wound should be visually inspected to establish:

1. the type and shape of wound

2. the depth – abrasion, skin deep through fatty tissue, or full thickness

3. evidence of whether any underlying structures are visible and whether they appear intact

4. any obvious foreign body

5. the nature of bleeding – bright red (arterial), or dark red (venous)

6. the severity of bleeding, particularly where blood is seen to 'spurt' in a pulsating manner.

A more detailed assessment by experienced staff will establish the degree of movement and sensation in the patient, in order to decide how to manage the wound.

X rays
Any wound involving glass should be X-rayed, unless there are no signs of a glass foreign body in situ. It is particularly important to consider X-rays for those who present with glass wounds after consuming alcohol

or drugs, because their sensory perception is reduced, and their account of events may be incomplete.

Covering the wound

While waiting a decision as to wound management, all wounds should be covered. If the patient is likely to be waiting a long time, then at least four layers of paraffin gauze dressing should be applied.

A dry piece of gauze should be placed on top of the paraffin gauze. This will keep the wound occluded, and reduce the risk of adhesion when the dressing is removed. Dry gauze alone tends to stick. This creates the risk of removing the epithelial cells around the wound, as well as creating additional bleeding when the dressing is removed.

Similarly, when you need to remove a dressing that has adhered to the skin, you should immerse the wound in saline. Continue the immersion until the layer of dressing nearest the wound soaks off without effort.

Elevating heavily bleeding wounds

Limbs with wounds that are bleeding heavily should be elevated. Apply direct pressure in an effort to slow the bleeding down.

Any foreign bodies in the wound should be brought to the attention of more experienced staff, before applying pressure over them, or trying to remove them.

Find out what methods are used to elevate limbs in the department, because methods vary. Possible techniques include

(a) Bradford slings
(b) high arm slings
(c) slings made from draw sheets attached to infusion stands.

For lower limbs, the patient can be positioned the wrong way round on the trolley, so as to use the head end to elevate the legs.

Pay particular attention to any wound around the trunk of the body, especially the chest or abdomen. Such wounds should immediately be referred to a more experienced member of staff.

Wound closure

Several products are available to achieve wound closure. However, it should be remembered that each wound is individual to the patient, who should be treated in a way appropriate to his or her needs.

The option to leave a wound exposed

Sometimes it is not practical to close a wound, or dress it. Those circumstances generally arise when:

▶ Small superficial wounds occur in the scalp, or in areas where skin creasing occurs such as around the eyelids or in the axilla.

▶ Superficial wounds are found to mucous membranes inside the mouth or around the genitalia.

▶ Multiple small cuts appear on the hand, such that the dressing of each wound would result in physical dysfunction for the patient. This has to be balanced against allowing those wound to heal conservatively.

▶ Most facial wounds.

Wound glue

Wound tissue adhesive provides an effective and relatively painless alternative to sutures. To apply the glue it is necessary to ensure that the skin is dry.

The only types of wounds suitable for wound glue are:

1. superficial or skin deep incisional lacerations
2. lacerations not involving the eye
3. lacerations not involving mucosa
4. lacerations that are not over the site of a joint
5. lacerations where the skin is not affected by disease.

Adhesive wound closures

These are linear paper strips with an adhesive backing. They are designed to be placed across the wound so as to close it. Patients know these devices as 'butterfly plasters'. They are so-called after the original winged version, which is not used as much today. Brand names such as steristrip and leucostrip are among others found on the shelves of most departments.

The same restrictions apply as with wound glue. Wounds over joints or deep wounds must not be dealt with using these devices, which are intended for superficial or skin deep lacerations only. Adhesive strips should always be applied in such a way that they are 'gated' so that they are secure during movement in all directions.

Wound staples

Wound staples are an option for managing superficial or skin deep lacerations on limbs, as opposed to the trunk, face or head. The cosmetic effect of staples means they should not be used on the face. Full thickness lacerations must still be dealt with using conventional sutures.

Make sure a staple remover is available for when the patient is to have the staples removed.

Sutures

The suturing of wounds would supply enough material for a book on its own. We can only offer an overview here. There are two types of sutures used in A&E:

1. absorbable – used to suture underlying structures
2. non-absorbable – used to suture skin.

Each suture is graded according to the thickness of the thread. This is denoted by a number followed by a forward slash and zero. The thickest thread available is 0/0, and the thinnest is 8/0.

Materials that sutures are made from vary, and the brand names even more. Absorbable sutures are normally made from material that is degradable over time, and non-absorbable ones from nylon or less commonly from silk. However, more and more synthetic materials are now being developed, advancing further the quality of suture material available.

As a junior nurse it is unlikely that you will be suturing wounds, but it is important that you know how to set a suture trolley up for a more experienced nurse or doctor, and to have a rough idea of the type of suture that you can provide.

Practical methods of wound closure

The stages of wound treatment

There are five stages to treating a wound in A&E:

1. giving appropriate pain relief
2. exploration of the wound
3. cleaning and irrigation of the wound

4. wound apposition and repair
5. providing an appropriate dressing and advice to the patient.

Appropriate pain relief

Oral analgesia may be appropriate before repairing wounds that do not require a local anaesthetic, but that have bruising and tenderness around the wound site.

Simple analgesia such as Paracetamol, given thirty minutes before treatment, may provide additional comfort during wound cleaning and repair.

Abrasions require scrubbing under local anaesthetic in order to remove dirt and avoid a tattoo effect which can arise if dirt is retained in the wound just under the superficial layers of the skin. The issue of anaesthesia is one that should be discussed with a more senior colleague because there is often a fine line between the amount of scrubbing that can be undertaken using local infiltration and larger wounds that may require a general anaesthetic. Topical anaesthetic gel is not within the terms of product licence for use directly onto skin wounds.

Local infiltration
Local infiltration with Lignocaine 1% to a maximum of 3mg per kg will provide adequate local anaesthesia. The 1% solution comes at a strength of 10mg per ml. A 70 kg adult could therefore have a maximum of 21mls. Solutions of 0.5% and 2% Lignocaine are also available, but 1% tends to be the most commonly used.

Digital nerve or ring blocks
Digital nerve or ring blocks are used when an entire digit has to be anaesthetised in order to repair the wound. They are also used in other situations, such as for pain relief in amputation, or when reducing dislocations. In ring block it is normal to use the drugs Marcain or Bupivocaine, either in isolation or in mixture with Lignocaine.

If a mixture is being drawn up, remember to obtain the Lignocaine first, if it comes from a bottle that may be needed for further doses later. This will prevent contamination of Lignocaine with Bupivocaine or Marcain for the next patient who may only require Lignocaine. Mixing in this way is also strictly speaking out of product licence.

Node blocks
Node blocks are used to anaesthetise the pathway of a specific nerve or

group of nerves. For example, this could be the ulna nerve which would incorporate the little finger and the medial aspect of the ring finger at any point distal to the point at which the anaesthetic was infiltrated.

Any local anaesthetic should be administered with the patient lying down on a couch. Thus, if the patient feels faint, they will not run the risk of falling and injuring themselves. For the same reasons all wound treatments should be carried out with the patient lying flat.

Exploration of the wound

Apart from checking to make sure there are no foreign bodies, exploration of wounds is better carried out by experienced staff. Evidence of tendon or muscle damage, and specific difficulties in managing rupture in blood vessels, need experience to ensure a good closure of the wound and a positive healing process.

The nurse closing the wound should always make a point of checking the function of the area concerned before and after treatment. Any pathology that might not have been obvious on initial assessment can then be identified and treated.

Cleaning and irrigation

Cleaning

All wounds need to be thoroughly cleaned before closure or dressing. Debate continues as to which solutions are most appropriate for wound cleaning. Normal saline is the most commonly used.

When cleaning a wound, the area of tissue underneath any flap wounds should be folded back so that the underside of the flap can be cleaned.

Irrigation

Irrigation of a wound is necessary where the wound is deep, and where debris may have entered the deeper layers underneath the wound. This is normally carried out by the use of a 20 ml syringe containing normal saline. A volume of at least 100 mls should be flushed through to irrigate properly.

Wound apposition and repair

Incisional wounds heal well when the two wound edges are equally apposed to each other, and where the method used to close the wound keeps it secure. Difficulties can arise when wounds involving skin loss need to be repaired.

In case of skin loss, an experienced member of staff should always be asked for advice. There may be options to partially close the wound, or allow the wound to heal by granulating from the bottom upwards. Wound glue and steristrips should not be applied over joints. Sutures should not be inserted into pre-tibial flap wounds, because the blood supply is insufficient to support sutures (unless a single holding suture is judged appropriate by a senior member of staff).

Facial wounds
Facial wounds and wounds to the lip and ears present different problems of a cosmetic, as well as clinical, nature. You should not be left to manage these types of wounds unsupervised.

Appropriate dressing and advice to the patient

As the debates go on about the most appropriate types of wound dressing, it would be impossible to specify particular dressings to use following wound repair. Dry dressings, non adhesive dressings, paraffin gauze dressings and many brand names that provide variations of those are available. Take time to find out what practice applies in your own department.

When a dressing is applied it should be secure but not constrictive. It should allow the patient as much function as possible within the physical limitations of the injury. Bandages should be secured with tape rather than a pin, especially in children.

Importance of wound advice
The wound advice given to patients is important for two reasons:

1. They need to know how to prevent complications in wound healing.
2. They need to recognise the signs of complications if they arise.

Preventing complications
Prevention of complications can be achieved by giving the following advice:

▶ Keep any dressing that may have been applied clean and dry.

▶ Don't lift weights through the injured limb during the initial period of healing.

▶ Take some gentle exercise through the natural range of movements, three or four times a day for ten minutes at a time. The exercise should be gentle in order to prevent stiffness in the affected area.

Signs of complications
Signs of complication in wound healing typically include:

1. abnormal pain or soreness around the wound site
2. yellow or green discharge through the dressing
3. general feeling of a raised temperature or malaise
4. tenderness in the lymph nodes proximal to the wound
5. excessive bleeding from the wound.

Summary

▶ A wound is a break in the continuity of the skin.
▶ Eight classifications of wound can occur in isolation or combination.
▶ All wounds need to be covered while the patient is in A&E.
▶ Exploration, cleaning and irrigation of all wounds is essential.
▶ Appropriate dressing and advice should be given in all cases.

Helping you learn

Progress questions
1. Describe four classifications of wound.
2. What structures would you expect to find underneath a wound to the finger?
3. What areas would not be appropriate for the use of staples in wound closure?

Seminar discussions
1. How extensive would you regard abrasions had to be before a general anesthetic is considered?
2. How would you deal with a wound that required sutures where the patient declined but said that they would accept steristrip?

3. What would you do with a wound that is bleeding heavily but that contains an obvious foreign body?

Practical assignment

Make a list of all the wound care products in your department. Ask your mentor to discuss their specific applications with you.

LRS: Somerset College

Medical Emergencies

One-minute summary – Collapse, chest pain, difficulty breathing, over-dose, gastro-intestinal bleeding and headaches are common presentations of medical emergency in A&E. Haematological conditions and established syndromes also contribute to this group but to a lesser extent. The most extreme medical emergency is that of cardiac and respiratory arrest. For this the Resuscitation Council (UK) guidelines should be followed. This means a logical team-based approach consistent with your own departmental policy. Priorities in dealing with medical emergencies begin with assessment of the airway breathing and circulation. This is followed by appropriate action if there is absence or compromise in any of those areas. A systematic assessment is then made of the primary presenting symptoms, moving on to observe more subtle signs that may indicate the investigations needed to reach a firm diagnosis.

In this chapter you will learn about the nursing management of:

▶ cardiac and respiratory arrest
▶ the unconscious patient
▶ collapse
▶ other medical emergencies.

Cardiac and respiratory arrest

It is necessary first of all to deal with the role that you would play in a cardiac/respiratory arrest. As this is the most extreme medical emergency it is often regarded as the most stressful by nursing and medical staff alike. If you feel apprehensive about dealing with your first arrest then take heart that your feelings are completely normal, and that with experience the situation will become less traumatic.

Patients in cardiac arrest present in one of three ways:

1. via the ambulance service with prior warning (usually only a few minutes)

2. by self presentation through other modes of transport such as friends or relatives

3. arresting while already present in the department.

As a junior nurse you would not be expected to play an advanced role in the management of cardiac arrest. It is however important that you are competent in two specific areas, namely that of recognising cardiac and respiratory arrest and, after raising the alarm, being able to perform chest compression as part of the team in the resuscitation room.

The signs of cardiac and respiratory arrest

▶ The patient is unconscious and is therefore unresponsive to painful stimuli.

▶ When the airway is opened there are no breath sounds and there is no evidence of the chest rising and falling after looking, listening and feeling for a maximum of 10 seconds.

▶ There is no palpable pulse at the carotid after feeling for a maximum of 10 seconds.

Managing cardiac and respiratory arrest
The official guidelines on basic life support are available in full from the Resuscitation Council (UK), the address of which is given at the end of this chapter. You should make a point of reading them thoroughly and making early efforts to do the basic life support course and to pass the assessments that go with it.

It is not possible to offer up-to-date guidance around the resuscitation guidelines that are produced by the Resuscitation Council (UK) given that they are under constant review. There should be an opportunity to undergo basic life support training as part of mandatory training within your department and the latest guidelines for basic life support in adults and children can be seen at the resuscitation council web site at *www.resus.org.uk*

In your first exposure to this situation there will hopefully be enough experienced staff on site very quickly to allow you the opportunity to watch and learn, perhaps keeping any questions back until the event has reached a conclusion.

Nursing roles in a cardiac arrest

Different departments will have specific roles for nursing medical and other staff in a cardiac arrest situation. Airway management and ventilation, intravenous access defibrillation and drug administration form the specialist interventions that accompany chest compressions during a cardiac arrest.

As stated earlier, it is not possible to present the latest Resuscitation Council (UK) guidelines in this publication due to the constant reviews that emerging new evidence brings. You are advised to seek advice from more senior staff in accessing the current policy within your department for the delivery of basic life support in so far as it would be considered to be your role in a cardiac arrest.

Drawing up drugs and infusions

The drugs required include Adrenaline in both 1mg and 5mg doses, Atropine in 1mg and 3mg doses, Lignocaine, and sodium bicarbonate solution 8.4% for use after blood gas measurement in prolonged resuscitation. It is also necessary to have a 500ml bag of normal saline or other crystalloid solution as a fluid chaser for the drugs. The nurse drawing up drugs should document the time that each drug is administered, and the time at which any defibrillation has been delivered, along with the number of joules given.

It is also important for the same nurse to note the rhythm displayed by the cardiac monitor before any pharmacological or electrical interventions. The start time and the time at which cardiac output returned, or at which the resuscitation was stopped, should also be recorded.

Defibrillation

Electrical chaos within the conducting system of the heart may produce ventricular fibrillation. Contraction of the heart muscle is not then possible. The only remedy for this situation is **defibrillation**. It is not within the scope of this guide to explore the algorithms that govern defibrillation. These can be found in the guidelines for advanced life support published by the Resuscitation Council (UK). The key aspect of defibrillation that applies to junior staff is to provide for your own safety when a defibrillator is in use.

▶ *Important note* – A defibrillator is a highly dangerous piece of equipment. If any person has contact with the patient, the person delivering the shock, the trolley or any appendage that attaches to the patient when a shock is due to be delivered, the same shock intended for the patient could be delivered to yourself with potentially <u>fatal consequences</u>. Before charging and delivering the DC shock a clear instruction will be given to 'stand clear'. It is vital that you do so, making sure that no part of yourself or your uniform is in contact with the patient, trolley or connecting equipment.

The management of relatives
This at first requires nursing staff with some experience because it will be likely that they will:

1. want to know what is happening
2. possibly want to be present in the resuscitation room.

If the opportunity presents itself, try to observe a more senior member of staff dealing with relatives. You will be able to take this role on as your experience increases. Most departments adopt a policy of being diplomatic and honest, and advocate the use of plain English when telling relatives what is happening. Despite natural pleas from relatives for predictions of outcome in such dire situations, it is wise to confine any information to the facts of what is happening at present. The issue of whether relatives are allowed to be present in the resuscitation room is one of departmental policy.

Other tasks
You will have to cut clothing through the length of both upper and lower arms in order to gain intravenous access, and to record a blood pressure should a cardiac output return.

The unconscious patient

Patients who are unconscious should be nursed in an area with appropriate resuscitation facilities. Most major A&E departments have a room dedicated to that purpose. In those departments which do not, it is essential to ensure that the patient is near to a reliable supply of oxygen and suction, and that the suction apparatus includes suction catheters. Airway adjuncts such as oropharangeal and nasal airways should be available.

Protection of the airway

▶ *Important note* – The movements of the patient described in this
   section do NOT apply in situations of trauma.

The patient should be turned onto his side in the recovery position, so
that gravity can play a natural part in protecting the airway. The
patient may need to be moved out of this position for the purpose of
examination later. Appropriate numbers of colleagues will be required
to help with moving the patient into this position.

If the airway is, or becomes, noisy then the following manoeuvres
should be attempted, remembering that you should call for immediate
help in any airway management situation:

1. Open the airway and apply gentle oropharangeal suction to
   remove excess saliva (if too vigorous this may induce vomiting).

2. Change the position of the head so that the neck is slightly more
   extended.

3. Gently perform a jaw thrust (Note 1).

4. Gently attempt to insert an oropharangeal airway after sizing it
   appropriately (Note 2). This may also induce vomiting; if so it
   must be removed immediately.

5. Call for help at this stage because more experienced staff will be
   needed to move the situation on.

   Note 1 – You will need to be shown in practice how to perform a jaw
   thrust because it is an important airway manoeuvre that cannot be
   learned from a textbook alone.

   Note 2 – An airway is the correct size when the phalange and the
   end of the airway correspond to the distance between the corner of
   the lip and the angle of the jaw when the airway is placed against
   the side of the patient's face.

The options for nasopharyngeal airways or a definitive airway through
intubation is not a decision to be taken at a junior level. This is why
help is required after completing the basic airway management as
detailed above.

When the airway has been stabilised it is important to establish
whether or not the patient has chronic obstructive pulmonary disease
(COPD) prior to the administration of oxygen which in non-COPD

patients should be delivered through a non-rebreathing mask at 10 12 litres. Immediate medical help is required in drowsy or unconscious patients who are suspected or known to have COPD.

All unconscious patients should have cardiac monitoring and pulse oxymetry. It is essential to record their neurological observations every 15 minutes and to document the findings on a neurological observation chart. Be careful with painful stimuli that you stay with sternal rubbing only. The pinching of earlobes or pressing on nail beds or other elaborate forms of painful stimuli are not acceptable. In extreme cases such practices could lead to legitimate allegations of assault.

All unconscious patients require a BM reading to determine their capillary blood sugar measurement. They also need a temperature reading to exclude infection or hypothermia. An ECG should be recorded at some stage to exclude a cardiac event that might have caused the collapse.

It is also likely that an arterial blood gas sample may be taken. In this case the nurse's role is to safely transfer the sample to the site of the nearest analysing machine, and apply direct pressure over the arterial puncture site for at least five minutes. In this way any bleeding can be minimised.

The cause of unconsciousness, the number of immediate radiological investigations and the accessibility of an in-patient facility will all determine how long the patient will remain the responsibility of A&E. However, unconscious patients should not be left unattended, and escorts should be provided for any transfer that takes place.

Never be afraid to ask for help when dealing with or supervising an unconscious patient. Experienced staff know how rapidly the conditions of such patients can change. They would not expect you to be able to offer accurate interpretation or action in that scenario.

Nursing management of 'collapse'

Strictly speaking, 'collapse' means that the patient falls to the floor through loss of consciousness. But the term is often used inappropriately. For example, arriving patients may have been found asleep on park benches due to alcohol consumption; they are checked into A&E as 'collapse' when there is no other convenient term to write on the A&E notes to explain their attendance. It is for this reason that an accurate history relating to the presentation is taken and carefully documented.

A handy mnemonic exists to provide you with a checklist of reasons for collapse:

A E I O U   T I P S
A   Asphyxia, asthma, anaphylaxis
E   Epilepsy
I   Ischaemia – cerebrovascular accident, transient ischaemic attack, cardiac event
O   Overdose, opiates
U   Uraemia – as in metabolic disturbances
T   Toxicity, trauma, temperature
I   Insulin (diabetes)
P   Psychiatric
S   Shock

Sometimes a patient will arrive in the department during the acute stages of the event. In those situations a diagnosis can be made quite easily. However there also situations where the event has moved on and the symptoms are less obvious. This is where the subsequent medical examination will look for more subtle signs that might lead to an accurate diagnosis.

The principles of airway and breathing assessment in cardiac arrest as described earlier apply to any patient who has collapsed, because failure to recognise those first two areas of priority will compromise any other interventions.

Other medical emergencies

In a publication such as this it is not possible to detail every condition found in a medical nursing textbook. The short paragraphs that follow are intended as an overview, hopefully with some important practical tips to help your management of these patients in A&E.

Asthma
Guidelines from the British Thoracic Society provide evidence of current best practice in the management of asthma in the UK. These guidelines can be viewed on their web site, the address for which is listed

in the section on web sites for nurses at the back of this book. Never underestimate the potential for asthma to result in the death of a patient. Although asthma is common there is no room for complacency when making an assessment of the asthmatic whether it be an adult or a child. Some points about asthma:

▶ Beware the silent asthmatic – the asthmatic too exhausted to talk needs very senior and immediate help.

▶ Severe attacks are accompanied by a rapid pulse (tachycardia).

▶ While reassuring the patient never say to an asthmatic, 'Now just relax and try to breath normally' because there is nothing that they would rather do than that if only it were physiologically possible.

▶ Try to get three peak flow readings with the best possible technique but don't persist if the patient is becoming exhausted or distressed. In that situation get senior help quickly.

▶ Nebulisers driven from an oxygen source require at least six litres of oxygen to work properly. Some departments may advocate nebulising patients over 40 years old on air to avert potential respiratory depression in chronic obstructive pulmonary disease (COPD). Find out what your local procedure is.

▶ After the completion of a nebuliser it is wise to wait at least ten minutes before repeating a peak flow reading, to allow the drugs time to work.

▶ All asthmatics should have their temperature recorded to exclude infection as the primary trigger.

▶ The usual first line drug regime in asthma is Nebulised Salbutamol (Ventolin) 2.5mg – 5mg, with or without Ipratropium bromide (Atrovent) 0.5mg and with the option to give a dose of intravenous hydrocortisone 100mg – 200mg which will help in the hours to come.

▶ The second line of treatment is with intravenous Aminophyline. This should never be administered quickly, or without cardiac monitoring in situ.

▶ If deterioration continues then a general anaesthetic followed by intubation and ventilation becomes an option.

Epilepsy

▶ Epileptic fits are localised or generalised, taking the form of petit mals or grand mals.

▶ Epileptics present either for the first time or as 'known' epiletics when the fits have been recognised as those of epilepsy.

▶ Epilepsy can be idiopathic (unknown) in origin, or due to a number of known causes.

▶ Status epilepticus is said to occur when there is continuous seizure activity or recurrent seizures lasting at least 30 minutes without the recovery of consciousness.

▶ Grand mal fits go through aura, tonic, clonic, and recovery phases.

▶ Support of the airway and protection from further injury are the two priorities in managing the initial period of convulsions.

▶ During the recovery phase the administration of oxygen through a non rebreathing mask at 10 – 12 litres will assist cerebral oxygenation.

Unresolving convulsions require the insertion of a cannula and the incremental administration of an intravenous muscle relaxant.

Diabetic emergencies

▶ Diabetics are diet, tablet or insulin dependent and when they present to A&E it is due to problems with either hypo- or hyperglycaemia.

▶ Hypoglycaemia usually results, not from a drop in blood sugar, but from the rate at which the blood sugar drops. A level of 2.2 – 2.8 is the marker for this state. Signs include headache and tremors with reduced concentration moving to sweating, tachycardia and coma. There may be irreversible cerebral damage if the state is not corrected.

▶ Correction of hypoglycaemia is urgent. The conscious patient can be given a drink of milk with glucose, which might be sufficient to reverse the state. Dextrose can also be given intramuscularly. Several preparations of this type exist.

▶ Hypoglycaemia where the patient is unable to drink requires the insertion of a cannula and the administration of 50ml of Dextrose 50%. Recovery is quite dramatic. A period of observation for an hour or so with a sweet drink and some food should be sufficient to have the patient go home with appropriate follow up either through outpatients or from the GP.

▶ Hyperglycaemia has a slower onset. It presents with a raised BM reading, extreme thirst, dehydration and a raised temperature. There will be glucose and ketones in the urine, a smell of ketones on the breath and an increase in urine output.

First line management is to insert a cannula. Blood samples are taken for a laboratory blood sugar, urea and electrolytes and a full blood count, along with blood cultures if the temperature is high. Arterial blood gas analysis is essential in determining how sick the patient is.

Fluid resuscitation is of the utmost importance. The fluid of choice is normal saline, but in the critically ill patient an initial bolus of colloid may be used. Intravenous Actrapid insulin is then given. The IV route is preferable since the patient will be peripherally shut down. An infusion of insulin is commenced in titration to the fall in blood sugar. All intravenous infusions must be placed on the same arm to allow the frequent blood tests to be taken from the other side.

▶ *Note* – The normal saline may also contain a potassium supplement because potassium is lost in the urine, but this should not be added to the initial resuscitation fluids unless the potassium level is known to be low. Particular care is needed in controlling the rate of any infusion containing potassium due to the risk of cardiac arrest if it is given too quickly, or in too high a dose.

Chest pain

Although cardiac pain needs to be considered in any patient presenting with chest pain, it should be remembered that there are many causes of chest pain. These include:

1. spontaneous pneumothrax – collapse of a portion of lung tissue

2. costocondritis – inflammation of the costal cartilage

3. pulmonary embolus – occlusion to the pulmonary circulation

4. pneumonia with pleurisy – inflammation of the lung involving the surrounding pleura

5. oesophagitis – erosion of the outer lining of the oesophagus.

Angina and myocardial infarction
Occlusion of the coronary artery will in most cases produce chest pain. If that occlusion is sufficiently severe then it will starve the myocardium (middle layer of heart muscle) of a blood supply sufficient to produce death of that portion of muscle and so a myocardial infarction has occurred.

During such an event enzymes are released into the blood stream. These can be measured to confirm the diagnosis. There are alterations in the electrical conduction of the heart, as demonstrable on an ECG. These changes are not necessarily immediate, so the decision as to whether a patient goes to a coronary care unit or to an acute medical ward is sometimes less than easy to make.

It is also important to stress that a 'silent myocardial infarction' can occur where no pain is experienced at all. Only symptoms of lethargy and dizziness present to A&E in a patient who suspects that nothing significant is wrong.

The presenting symptoms of a myocardial infarction are:

(a) central crushing severe chest pain – occasionally abdominal pain may be present

(b) the pain sometimes radiates to the jaw or through the neck down the left arm

(c) retrosternal pain is significant in myocardial infarction

(d) feelings of nausea or vomiting

(e) dyspnoea, sweating and tachycardia.

A combination of these symptoms if left to deteriorate untreated will produce a state of inadequate tissue perfusion (shock) and cardiogenic shock will develop.

Nursing care of a patient with a possible myocardial infarction

Note – Never attempt to deal with one of these patients on your own.

1. Establish that the patient does not have chronic obstructive pulmonary disease (COPD) and administer high flow oxygen

through a non-rebreathing mask.

2. Attach the patient to a cardiac monitor.

3. Establish pulse oxymetry.

4. Take a blood pressure on the opposite arm to the one that has the pulse oxymetry probe.

5. Take an ECG.

6. Record a temperature, respiratory rate and BM reading.

7. Assist with cannulation and the taking of blood samples.

8. Administer soluble aspirin 300mg orally to start thrombolysis if prescribed.

9. Draw up requested analgesia, normally Diamorphine 2.5mg – 5mg IV, preceded by 10mg Metochlopramide IV as an anti emetic followed by a flush of normal saline.

10. Continue close monitoring of the patient until transferred to a coronary care unit.

Angina is slightly different in terms of management. For patients with known angina it may be appropriate to give glyceryl trinitrate sublingually (under the tongue) or a slower released nitrate tablet of Buccal suscard to a maximum dose of 5mg placed between the surfaces of the gums to absorb slowly. Glyceryl trinitrate may cause a sudden drop in blood pressure which can result in a fainting episode. If this fails to alleviate the pain then Diamorphine can be given as described above. Unstable angina requires admission to an acute medical ward or CCU for observation and stabilisation and a 9th infusion may be required.

Some A&E departments will start a nitrate infusion before transfer to the ward or CCU.

Cerebrovascular accident (CVA) & transient ischaemic attack (TIA)

The difference between a CVA and a TIA is only the duration of the symptoms. In a TIA these will pass to a stage of complete recovery within 24 hours of the event. The extent of neurological pathology that a TIA is able to generate can be severe and by the same token a CVA can be very mild in the dysfunction that it produces.

Even for the unconscious patient – where hearing is the last sense to go and the first to return – it is essential to provide reassurance in this frightening time. Remember, the patient has no choice but to put himself into the hands of nursing and medical staff to provide for even his most basic needs.

The degree of neurological impairment will depend on the side of the brain and the extent of damage to the area of the brain affected. The side on the body affected will be opposite to the affected side of the brain below the level of the neck. A weakness down the left arm will originate from a cerebral lesion on the right side of the brain.

Neurological impairment can include

hemiparesis/hemiplegia	weakness / paralysis on one side of the body
dysphasia	difficulty speaking
aphasia	inability to speak
dysphagia	difficulty swallowing.

Good basic nursing care is paramount in patients who have sustained a CVA. This is because of their vulnerability to pressure sores and their basic needs for eating, drinking and dealing with the needs of their bladder and bowel.

Take some time to identify what type of pressure relieving devices are used in your department. These may include pressure-relieving mattresses, and protocols for turning and managing pressure areas. A scale or model may be used to assess the risk of pressure sores.

There may be specific documentation for noting the action to be taken in respect of these important aspects of basic nursing care. Make sure that limbs are in a comfortable position and not crushed by body pressure. Although movement may not be possible there may still be some feeling remaining or returning. Cast your mind back to when you last woke up with 'pins & needles' down one arm; you will have some inkling of the need for correct positioning of the patient on the A&E trolley.

Mouth care is essential for any patient who is unable to drink or who has been vomiting. Most departments have small mouth care packs, the same as those found on the wards when you had your placements earlier in your training.

It is important to take time to communicate with patients who are conscious. You will be the person most exposed to them in A&E. Their memories of A&E will depend as much on the quality of your communication with them, as on how well you delivered technical care.

Overdose

Overdose is the consumption of a drug or drugs in excess of the recommended dose. Patients with overdose present in one of three ways:

1. accidental unintentional ingestion through self administration or genuine error

2. deliberate ingestion with the intention to harm or kill themselves

3. overdose secondary to the malicious act of a third party (attempted murder).

Common drugs used in overdose:

1. analgesics such as Paracetamol, Aspirin, Tylex, and Naproxen
2. tricyclic antidepressants such as Amitriptyline, Nortriptyline, and Prothiden
3. benzodiazepine antidepressants such as Diazipam
4. opiates, especially IV heroin (Diamorphine)
5. Seratonin reuptake inhibitors such as Prozac.

The history that you elicit from the patient or accompanying personnel should include:

▶ what was taken
▶ how much
▶ at what time and in what stages
▶ with or without alcohol
▶ what symptoms have been present prior to presenting at A&E.

It needs to be remembered that intentional overdose has two components of care. The physical component of treating the effects that the drugs will have on the body takes priority in all cases but the second and equally important aspect is the intent behind the act of taking the overdose in the first place. Deliberate self harm is covered in Chapter 12 on psychiatric emergencies.

To manage the physical effects of the overdose the care that would apply to a patient who has collapsed or a patient who is unconscious would apply accordingly. Advice on specific management of poisoning can be obtained from a network of national poison information centres the telephone number for which will be available in your department. These numbers are not available to the public. There is also an internet facility through such databases as 'Toxbase' which is run by the Edinburgh poisons centre for which corporate access is pre-arranged and password protected.

The management of overdose is more conservative than it used to be. Oral emetics are no longer used. Activated charcoal is a more frequent treatment of choice. It is available in several makes. The adult dose is 50g and the dose in children calculated on a basis of 0.5 to 1g per kg of body weight.

Gastric lavage

The use of **gastric lavage** is still indicated in certain situations, and for that reason the procedure is worth explaining. Gastric lavage in children is now very rarely undertaken. Diagnostic drugs are available to temporarily displace the effects of opiates and Benzodiazepines. Those drugs are Naloxone (Narcan) and Flumazanil (Anexate).

The public imagine is of gastric lavage to be a 'stomach pump'. In fact no pump action is involved at all. The principle is that water is passed through a funnel down a tube that has been placed via the mouth through to the opening of the stomach. Then, by lowering the tube and funnel to the ground, the water – along with the gastric contents – drains out by natural gravity.

Gastric lavage needs to be carried out:

▶ with the patient's full informed consent

▶ in an environment that has a reliable source of oxygen and suction

▶ on a trolley that is capable of tilting the head downwards

▶ by at least two competent qualified nurses and a third person to support the position of the patient during the procedure

▶ in an environment where senior medical help is immediately available if required.

A trolley containing the following equipment should be made available:

a funnel
22mm gastric lavage tube
lubricating jelly
blue litmus paper
a supply of tepid water sufficient for at least 5 litres
a bucket
suction.

This procedure if carried out forcibly is not only unethical but physically dangerous. When you consider the precautions taken with endoscopy, one can see that risks of bleeding and trauma to the GI tract apply to gastric lavage in exactly the same way. Gastric lavage should never be seen as a punitive procedure.

It should not be attempted on any patient with the following conditions (for which medical help should be sought):

▶ peptic ulceration
▶ hiatus hernia
▶ trachiostomy or previous surgery to the throat excluding tonsillectomy as a child
▶ patients who become unduly short of breath when lying down
▶ where the patient is not sufficiently conscious to produce a good gag reflex.

Adopting a three-nurse procedure, the most experienced nurse should pass the tube. The second nurse should maintain suction to the mouth, and the third should support but not restrain the patient's arms.

After explaining the procedure to the patient, obtaining verbal consent and removing any dentures, the patient should be invited to lie on his left side with both arms behind him. Reassurance is the key to this procedure. Remember, the patient will find it frightening and invasive. Prior to tilting the patient the gastric lavage tube should be placed in front of him to measure the distance between the mouth and just below the diaphragm. This distance can then be compared with the incremental markers on the lavage tube, to estimate the distance required for the tube to pass.

The head of the trolley is tipped downwards to 45 degrees and the patient is asked to open his mouth. After a brief inspection to exclude any food or debris in the mouth the tube, the top of which has been lightly coated with lubricant jelly, is passed gently to the back of the throat. The patient is then told to swallow hard, and to keep swallowing. If the patient should vomit then the tube should be withdrawn and suction applied to keep the airway clear before re-inserting the tube.

When the tube is passed the funnel should be put to the ground. The gastric contents can then drain into the bucket. The litmus paper should catch the initial drainage in order to ensure that a now pink piece of litmus indicates that the contents from the tube are coming from the stomach. Some departments advocate taking a sample of contents at this stage in case the patient should die and some analyses of the contents might be necessary. This is not an established practise in all departments.

At this stage water can be placed in the funnel and passed down the tube, allowing time to reach the stomach before siphoning out. Large quantities of water should be avoided because it will induce vomiting. To fill a funnel initially to three quarters capacity is quite sufficient.

After the tube is clear of drugs activated charcoal, if prescribed, is placed gently into the stomach via the tube. When withdrawing the tube suction should be readily available and the patient should keep his mouth wide open so that a firm but even rate of withdrawal can take place. The patient should be offered a mouthwash after gastric lavage and any dentures should be returned.

Headaches

With the exception of trauma and pyrexia there are several groups of illness that present to A&E with headaches:

Tension headache

Muscles in the scalp have become strained and experience spasm that produces pain in the head and back of the neck. A tension headache is not associated with photophobia and treatment is through simple analgesia and rest. These are the most common types of headaches presenting to A&E.

Migraine

Thought to be due to spasm in the arterial vessels of the brain. It is more common in females than males and peaks in incidence in early adulthood. The headache is throbbing and severe and can be one sided and often preceded by visual changes such as flashing lights. Nausia, photophobia and vomiting are common and a severe migraine may produce neurological features similar to a transient ischaemic attack (TIA) as described earlier. Treatment is with an analgesia such as Paracetamol. Drugs such as Codeine Phosphate, which when given intramuscularly as a 60mg injection (1ml), is a controlled drug. It is usual to prescribe an anti emetic also since nausea is often a prominent symptom.

Temporal arteritis

This is due to inflammation over the temporal artery the causes of which are not clear. However it is only found in older people. This headache is normally local to the affected side, and there is marked swelling and tenderness over the affected artery. Treatment is with analgesics and steroids. In severe cases blindness can be induced if the vessels that supply the optic nerves become thrombosed or occluded.

Glaucoma
See ophthalmic emergencies.

Sinusitis
See ENT emergencies.

Subarachnoid haemorrhage
Bleeding into the subarachnoid space is normally due to a cerebral aneurysm or secondary to a head injury. The patient experiences a sudden, very severe headache (the worst in his life) and the level of consciousness may fall. The neurological signs will depend on the extent of the bleed which is diagnosed by a CAT or MRI scan. This condition is more common in younger adults.

Headaches with pyrexia
Encephalitis is a term used to describe an inflammatory process within the brain tissue. It is not within the scope of a short textbook such as this to provide detail in that area.

Meningitis is an inflammation of the meninges and hence of the cerebrospinal fluid that travels around the meninges to nourish the cells in the brain and also extends down the spinal cord. The cause can be either viral or, more seriously, bacterial and the signs and symptoms are:

▶ pyrexia > 37.0 degrees
▶ headache
▶ neck stiffness
▶ photophobia
▶ rash to the body that does not blanch under pressure
▶ nausea and sometimes vomiting.

If you are presented with a patient that displays the symptoms listed above then do not waste time taking clinical observations. Get senior nursing help immediately and observe how more experienced nursing and medical staff deal with the situation.

Their management will include:

1. taking universal precautions
2. inserting a cannula
3. taking blood for U&E FBC and blood cultures
4. administering oxygen
5. BM measurement
6. administering intravenous antibiotics immediately
7. administering intravenous fluids if signs of shock are present
8. transferring the patient to an appropriate ward or unit.

Gastrointestinal bleeding

The oesophagus, stomach, duodenum, small and large intestine, rectum and anus form the gastrointestinal tract. Gastrointestinal problems usually present to A&E in the form of abdominal pain, haematemasis (vomiting blood), or the passing of altered blood (malaena) or bright red blood from the rectum.

The line between medical and surgical conditions in this area is a very thin one because some of the conditions will be treated medically and some surgically. The decision will depend on the degree of bleeding, the age of the patient, and how well the patient may tolerate an anesthetic without prior treatment to stabilise the condition. It also depends on how certain the diagnosis is, given that clinical examination, blood tests and X-rays may be all there is to provide evidence of a firm diagnosis in the A&E setting.

Haematemasis

Vomiting blood is a serious symptom that should prompt you to look at the general condition of the patient for signs of hypovolaemic shock. These include:

▶ pale in colour
▶ sweating and cold to the touch
▶ tachycardia
▶ rapid shallow respiration
▶ low blood pressure (hypotension)
▶ thirst
▶ confusion or agitation
▶ capillary refill > 2 seconds.

In these symptoms urgent senior intervention is indicated. The patient should be in an area with good resuscitation facilities. High flow oxygen should be delivered via a non re-breathing mask along with pulse oxymetry, cardiac monitoring and an initial manual blood pressure. This should be followed by attachment to a machine that will generate frequent blood pressure readings at least every five minutes.

The patient should be kept warm. After a cannula has been secured, and blood samples taken, it may be appropriate to provide analgesia (usually morphine) if the blood pressure is high enough to support it. Intravenous colloid or crystalloid fluids will be established. O negative, type specific, or cross-matched blood will be given depending on the response to initial fluid resuscitation (usually one and a half litres of crystalloid). A nasogastric tube should be passed and if time permits a urinary catheter may be requested. An ECG should be taken to exclude the event leading to a myocardial infarction and the patient should then be transferred out of A&E to an appropriate ward, intensive care unit, or theatre, as appropriate.

The causes of haematemasis include perforation of gastric or duodenal ulceration, carcinoma of the stomach, and oesophageal varices. It may also occur after repeated vomiting, causing a tear in the lower oesophagus.

Haemoptysis is when the patient is coughing blood. The management is the same if there are signs of hypovolaemic shock. It is important to know how much a patient has coughed or vomited. Markers such as 'a teaspoonful' or 'a cupful' are often used as gauges in estimating the volume of blood lost.

Haematological conditions

Sickle cell crisis This is probably the only haematological disorder likely to present as a problem in its own right. Most other disorders present as a secondary problem for the patient, as in haemophilia. Here, the patient may have sustained a laceration as the primary cause of him being in A&E, yet the haemophilia still requires treatment as a result.

Sickle cell anaemia is a form of anaemia where the shape of the red blood cell is abnormal. This affects the uptake of oxygen and creates a thrombosis in the capillaries. The disorder is exclusive to Afro-Caribbeans. There is no definitive treatment to prevent symptoms permanently, except to transfuse in cases of severe anaemia.

In sickle cell crisis, the patient complains of severe muscle pain and dyspnoea (shortness of breath). It is important to give high flow oxygen and adequate opiate analgesia before referring the patient to the haematology team on call.

Other haematological disorders include:

haemophilia	Insufficient production of factor V111.
Von Willebrand's disease	As for haemophilia but with purpura of the skin.
Christmas disease	Insufficient production of factor IX.

Heart failure

This results from left ventricular failure where the lung is congested with fluid.

The physiology is complex. In brief, left ventricular failure occurs when the pressure in the left atrium and pulmonary veins rises due to failing of the ventricle as in myocardial infarction, obstruction as in aortic stenosis or due to an increased volume of blood to be handled due to aortic incompetence. An initial period of coping will give way to oedema and symptoms that include:

▶ dyspnoea
▶ the patient is pale in colour
▶ the patient is cold, clammy and sweaty to the touch
▶ the patient shows confusion and agitation
▶ there is low oxygen saturation.

In A&E it is anecdotally experienced that many of these patients in left ventricular failure present very early in the morning, just towards the end of a night shift. The fact that the care is labour-intensive makes it quite arduous at times. This may occur because the lungs become more congested when the patient lies flat.

Treatment is as follows:

▶ Keep the patient sitting well up.
▶ Administer high flow oxygen.
▶ Establish pulse oxymetry and cardiac monitoring.
▶ Produce a baseline set of observations including a BM reading.
▶ Take an ECG.
▶ Assist with securing the cannula and draw up IV drugs. These will include:

Diamorphine 2.5mg-5mg.

Metochlopramide 10mg.

Frusimide 50 – 100mg (10mg per ml).

Buccal Suscard 2mg-5mg between the gums.

Antibiotics if pyrexial (IV).

Salbutamol – if the patient has a wheeze,
but not in pure left ventricular failure.

▶ Intubation and mechanical ventilation may be necessary.

▶ Provide a warm blanket and keep the patient warm if not pyrexial.

▶ Assist with collection of arterial blood gas sample.

▶ A urinary catheter may be necessary.

▶ A chest X-ray will be taken at some stage.

▶ Transfer to appropriate care either in an intensive/coronary care unit or on a medical ward.

Care of the elderly in A&E

Like the rest of the NHS population the elderly generate a substantial workload within A&E. As pressure on resources continues to increase, the amount of care and expectation within the A&E field becomes ever greater.

Investment in good basic nursing care for the elderly in A&E will produce a potentially better outcome in the longer term. It will increase the number of patients with successful outcomes from in-patient care, and who will ultimately achieve discharge more quickly.

The following points should be considered when nursing the elderly within A&E:

▶ Dignity, kindness and respect are three things that any individual has a right to expect at all times.

▶ Pressure areas need to be monitored using any tools that your department has available.

▶ Toileting needs to be carried out on request. Any sites of injury need to be carefully accounted for during assistance with toileting procedures.

▶ Make full use of any aids that are available to you for moving and handling, for example slides, hoists, and slings.

▶ Food and drink is important if a long wait is in prospect and if fasting is not required.

▶ Mouth care should be given to those who can't eat and drink and to those with conditions that produce vomiting.

Summary

1. Several modes of presentation exist commonly in patients with medical emergencies.

2. Cardiac and respiratory arrest are the most extreme conditions presenting as a medical emergency.

3. The term 'collapse' is used to describe any patient who has endured a sudden onset of losing consciousness and falling to the floor, however the term is also abused when there seems no obvious adjective to describe the events leading to presentation in A&E.

4. Care needs to be taken in the assessment of asthma so that the 'silent' asthmatic is seen immediately.

5. In CVA/TIA, the unconscious and the elderly, communication is as vital as clinical procedures.

6. Signs of hypovolaemic shock are important to recognise in patients who are vomiting or coughing blood.

Resuscitation guidelines

Resuscitation Council (UK)
5th Floor
Tavistock House North
Tavistock Square
London WC1H 9HR

Helping you learn

Progress questions

1. Name three causes of collapse.

2. How long after a nebuliser should an asthmatic be left before taking a post peak flow reading?

3. What symptoms might you expect to see in sickle cell crisis?

Seminar discussions

1. A 95 year old man is brought to A&E because he is vomiting blood. The ambulance crew say that he has an inoperable carcinoma of the stomach. He goes into cardiac arrest. Do you attempt to resuscitate him?

2. How would you persuade a diabetic patient who has just recovered from a hypoglycaemic attack to visit their GP when the patient shrugs it all off as a minor issue?

3. A patient with clinical signs of hypovolaemic shock refuses to let you cut his clothing. How would you deal with this?

Practical assignments

1. Find the ECG machine in your department. Ask a senior member of staff to show you how to record an ECG.

2. Take time to examine the equipment in the resuscitation room.

Management of Trauma

One-minute summary – Managing trauma – multiple life-threatening injuries and shock – requires a logical team-based approach. The nursing and medical teams need to communicate effectively. Success is achieved by tackling the patient's problems in sequence – airway with cervical spine immobilisation, breathing, circulation, disability and examination for lesser injury. To begin with, the junior nurse will take and record serial observations and document the patient's property. With experience you will be able to perform other roles such as drug administration, log-rolling and physical treatments for each individual case.

In this chapter you will learn about:

▶ preparation for receiving the trauma patient
▶ initial stages of managing the airway
▶ common major injuries and their diagnosis
▶ burns and scalds
▶ the nursing role in major injuries.

Preparation for receiving the trauma patient

There are many situations that can produce major trauma. These include road traffic accidents, industrial accidents, assaults, accidents in the home or in the sporting arena. Whatever the cause, there is likely to be at least a few minutes warning of the patient's arrival, probably by ambulance.

This time is vital for preparation. It allows a chance for the right personnel and equipment to be ready when the patient arrives.

The structure of the team will vary according to the resources and structure of the department. You will certainly need to learn how to put out a call for a trauma team, and know who to expect will arrive to form that team.

As well as senior nurses and doctors from A&E, it may also be the practice to call for initial assistance from an anaesthetist and an operating department practitioner to be primarily responsible for airway management. While it is important to have the correct team present, it is just as important that other people do not get in their way. So if you are asked simply to observe, you will be asked to do so from a position away from the immediate area of the patient.

Equipment

The following equipment will need to ready for the patient's arrival:

▶ a trolley capable of tilting and accommodating X ray cassettes underneath the main chassis, plus oxygen and suction apparatus for transfer to destinations outside of A&E

▶ warm blankets – trauma patients become cold very easily and warm blankets help the peripheral circulation

▶ oxygen, suction and anaesthetic equipment

▶ cardiac monitor, pulse oxymetry and blood pressure recording facilities

▶ wide bore cannuli, tape to secure the cannuli and bandages

▶ blood bottles and forms for U&E, sugar, FBC, group and cross-matching

▶ universal precautions taken by all of the team of wearing aprons, gloves and goggles if appropriate

▶ a room and appropriate member of staff to accommodate any relatives.

Most patients who present by ambulance arrive already strapped to a spinal board. However, a spinal board should be available just in case.

Managing the airway

An immediate priority is management of the patient's airway, cervical spine, breathing and circulation.

Care in the resuscitation room usually begins with transferring the patient on the spinal board from the ambulance trolley to the A&E trolley, with the person at the head controlling the sequence of transfer.

The first few minutes of care for the trauma patient are very intensive. Despite the sense of urgency, it is important that a logical system is followed. Life threatening problems are dealt with as soon as they are discovered, following the systematic sequence of assessment that begins with checking the airway.

Airway problems

Without an obvious airway the patient could not breathe for himself. He could die from hypoxia very quickly.

This is why airway management is top of the agenda for the trauma patient. However, in trauma the airway is always managed along with protecting the cervical spine; a spinal cord injury caused through movement of the neck could result in death or paralysis. Hence the ambulance crew will have applied an appropriately sized semi-rigid neck collar at the scene.

In major trauma the airway should never be a junior nurse's responsibility. However, you should be aware of the likely sequence of events if the patient is unable to support his own airway.

Intubation

In major trauma a decision is very often made to intubate the patient early, because:

▶ the patient is unconscious

▶ there is clinical evidence of hypoxia – the patient is pale, clammy, sweating and dyspnoeic

▶ there is airway obstruction

▶ there are facial injuries that may cause oedema later on.

If intubation is going to be performed, the patient will usually be given a general anaesthetic very quickly first of all. If intravenous access has not been established in the pre-hospital environment, then two lines will be set up. We will deal with this in the section on circulation.

Action prior to intubation

Prior to intubating the patient, two things need to happen:

1. If the patient is to be anaesthetised the appropriate drugs need to be prepared and administered. These will include an induction agent.

2. Having induced anaesthesia a paralysing agent will be needed.

Following administration of these drugs the patient is both anaesthetised and paralysed. He is now completely dependent on the anaesthetist for his airway and breathing.

Oxygenation takes place through a bag-valve mask for at least 30 seconds. Then, an entotracheal tube is passed through the mouth into the trachea. It is secured through the inflation of a cuff around the tube and through securing the tube with a tie around the patient's face.

Endotracheal tubes vary in size between male and female patients. A male requires a tube size between 8.0mm and 9.0mm and a female one between 7.5mm and 8.5mm. The tube is then attached to an anaesthetic circuit so that ventilation can be controlled. The medical staff will check that the endotracheal tube is correctly placed by listening at the base of both lung fields. Conscious patients should be given high flow oxygen via a non-rebreathing mask. The use of oropharyngeal airways is only a holding measure pending a definitive airway achieved through oral endotracheal intubation.

Nasal endotracheal intubation, and the use of nasopharyngeal airways, are not recommended in trauma. This is due to the risk of causing trauma to the upper airway or creating complications in a base of skull fracture.

Suction of the airway is important in case secretions gather. This should take no more than 30 seconds using a suction catheter of appropriate size. Take time to study the sizes available. You will then be able judge what size to use for passing through the opening of an endotracheal tube or an oropharyngeal airway.

Breathing problems

Assessment of breathing is carried out once the patient's airway has been established. In practise, assessment of airway and breathing is done at about the same time. When assessing breathing, the following points will be observed:

1. respiratory rate
2. volume
3. rhythm

4. equality between both sides of the chest
5. excluding signs of paradoxical breathing.

Hypoxia is the main reason for breathing difficulties. Causes for a patient failing to breathe effectively include:

► tension pneumothorax
► pneumothorax
► cardiac tamponade
► flail chest
► aortic vessel rupture
► foreign body obstructing the lower airway
► hypovolaemia to the extent that respiratory arrest occurs.

It is very important to obtain a respiratory rate for recording onto the neurological observations chart. Not only does this give an indication of mechanical respiratory function, but in a patient with rapid and weak respirations there may be signs of hypovolaemic shock.

The injuries listed above that are included in the causes of breathing difficulties will be dealt with in the section on major injuries later in this chapter.

Circulation problems

Major trauma patients are threatened by an insufficient circulation of blood for adequate tissue perfusion. If the red cells that carry oxygen to the tissues become depleted through haemorrhage, then inadequate tissue perfusion will be the result. This state is known as 'shock'.

Physiological changes occur at tissue and cell level in shock and they include:

1. increase in heart rate
2. reduction in blood pressure
3. diversion of the blood supply to the major organs such as the lungs and the brain
4. peripheral circulation reduced producing poor capillary refill, sweating, cold and clammy skin and a pale complexion
5. reduction and eventually loss of consciousness
6. metabolic acidosis due to anaerobic metabolism at cellular level
7. end organ failure leading to cardiac and respiratory arrest.

Shock occurring in this way is called hypovolaemic shock. In A&E there two other types of shock that can present, cardiogenic shock and distributive shock:

▶ Cardiogenic shock arises out of cardiac compromise (see the chapter on medical emergencies).

▶ Distributive shock includes shock from anaphylaxis and burns, dealt with in the last section of this chapter.

In reality, clinical signs of shock may be delayed, due to a period of compensation that precedes the deleterious pathway of symptoms described above. In this period the baseline observations may be normal, giving a false impression that all is well. The compensation period in children is greater than in adults.

When making an assessment of the circulation, clear measurements must be taken of the level of consciousness. As a first step this can be done using the AVPU method of scoring:

    A   alert
    V   responds to verbal stimuli
    P   responds to painful stimuli
    U   unconscious

This very brief scoring, carried out by the medical staff, will develop rapidly into the documentation laid out on the Glasgow coma charts described in the chapter on observations.

Another way of detecting hypovolaemic shock is with the pulse pressure. This is calculated by measuring the blood pressure and subtracting the diastolic figure from the systolic figure. For example, in a blood pressure of 120/80 the pulse pressure is 120 − 80 which = 40mmHg. It is thought that a pulse pressure below 15mmHg indicates hypovolaemia.

The first blood pressure reading in a trauma patient should be taken manually, not automatically. This is because we cannot detect audible irregularities in the blood pressure with automatic machines. Also, machines are fallible and can yield inaccurate readings even in the best of circumstances.

Assessing circulation in trauma will include evaluating the baseline observations. Therefore it is vital that, within five minutes of the patient arriving in the resuscitation room, you have readings on:

1. level of consciousness
2. pulse
3. blood pressure
4. respirations

5. capillary refill
6. pupil size and reaction
7. BM reading.

Having assessed the circulation, the team must act on symptoms that may indicate hypovolaemia. If a patient is suffering from hypovolaemia due to blood loss from trauma, the only sure way to stop the bleeding is to 'turn off the tap' at source. But a decision for early surgical intervention has to be weighed against the certainty with which the source of bleeding can be identified, the likely success of surgery, and the ability of the patient to reach the operating theatre without further stabilisation. In the past the tendency has been to provide large volumes of fluid, to try and restore circulating volume.

Some physicians still favour fluids in large quantities, but many others now prefer to administer one and a half litres of warmed crystalloid fluid, such as Hartmans (compound sodium lactate). They then follow up with red cells in the form of whole blood, preferably of the type cross-matched to that of the patient. The theory is that to administer large quantities of fluid will only increase the pressure of blood (and hence red cell) loss, and therefore the circulating volume continues to be poor – not only in volume but in red cells as well.

Using whole blood at an early stage will replace red cells and provide a better holding measure in lieu of surgical intervention.

Before administering fluids it is necessary to ensure that two secure intravenous lines exist to carry the fluids and drugs. In some cases these will already have been inserted by the ambulance crew at the scene. In this case you will need to document the fluids given at the scene, as well as those given in the resuscitation room, on a fluid balance chart. Blood samples will be taken for:

▶ urea and electrolytes
▶ blood sugar
▶ full blood count
▶ group and cross matching
▶ pregnancy test in a female patient.

It is important to ensure that the fluids continue running to time. As the nurse responsible for making observations every 15 minutes, you must also watch the fluid administration and make it known when fluids are running out.

The final measure in maintaining circulation is to keep the patient warm with blankets. Trauma patients become cold very quickly, especially when several examinations and procedures are taking place at once.

Common major injuries and their diagnosis

Life threatening injuries need to dealt with immediately. When an assessment of the airway is being performed, and such a condition is discovered, that condition must be treated before moving on to the next stage of assessment. Listed below are these injuries and their treatments:

Pneumothorax

This is the collapse in the portion of a lung due to air entering the pleural cavity. This cavity, lying between the chest wall and the lung, usually has a negative pressure but air entry to the cavity converts this to positive pressure, which in turn causes a proportional part of the lung to collapse.

This in turn will create difficulty breathing. There is potential respiratory compromise if it is not treated. Treatment is by means of an intercostal drain, the procedure for which is outlined in the next section of this chapter. A rupture of blood vessels in the chest can produce the same phenomenon with blood. This is referred to as a haemothorax.

Tension pneumothorax

This is where a pneumothorax so massive has occurred, that the affected lung has collapsed completely, with a sufficiently high pressure of air to push the opposite lung into collapse. It is diagnosed through increasingly rapid respirations and dullness on the affected side. The primary symptom is the physical deviation of the trachea away from the affected side. This is imminently threatening to life. It requires the immediate insertion of a canula through the chest wall into the pleural space. This is a high risk, but potentially life saving manoeuvre, which will only be attempted by a very experienced clinician. It is for this reason that the procedure for this intervention is not detailed in this text. This procedure is also seen as a holding measure prior to a formal inter costal drain being inserted.

Cardiac tamponade

This is the term used to describe bleeding into the pericardial sack. This is life threatening because the myocardium cannot contract effectively if it is restricted by the presence of blood.

The cause for this is usually either direct trauma, as in stab wounds, or trauma to the upper abdomen where cardiac injury has occurred as part of a wider injury. Signs of cardiac tamponade include tachycardia, low blood pressure, and an enlargement of the neck veins.

Treatment is by means of pericardial aspiration. A spinal needle is inserted through the pericardium to aspirate the blood. This will require a dressing trolley and pack with some skin cleansing solution, plus a 20ml syringe and a dry dressing with some tape and a good source of light.

Head injury

Head injury needs to be thought of as 'brain injury'. The cranium is an inflexible container for the brain tissue and vascular supply. Trauma to the skull will produce a movement of the brain rather like a jelly on a plate. For this reason the damage is often sustained at the opposite side to the site of direct trauma, producing what is called a 'contra coup' (counter blow) injury.

The surface of the brain is protected by fibrous linings. These comprise the pia mater, dura mater, arachnoid mater, and subarachnoid mater. Bleeding and haemotoma formation is possible at any point between these linings. Since brain cells do not regenerate, the management of head injury is focussed on preventing secondary injury. The detail of head injury management is covered in the chapter on surgical emergencies.

Thoracic injury

This is immediately life threatening. The injuries of pneumothorax, tension pneumothorax, and cardiac tamponade have already been discussed. However, other injuries to the thorax need considering.

Flail chest, for example, is the condition where three or more ribs on the same side have sustained fractures at more than one point. This produces 'paradoxical breathing'. Here, the segment involved rises on expiration and falls on inspiration, the opposite to the normal mechanics of respiration. Large flail segments create insufficient function in respiration, and so it is necessary to intubate and ventilate the patient.

Aortic vessel rupture, if it occurs, is often difficult to diagnose – especially if other hypovolaemic injuries are present. Unequal pulses when radial and femoral pulses are compared may be one of very few symptoms to suggest aortic rupture.

In the absence of a spinal cord injury there can be paralysis below the level of rupture which may lead to a suspicion of aortic rupture. A surgical repair is the only definitive treatment is this injury.

Abdominal injuries

Extending from the diaphragm to the pelvis, the abdomen comprises the lower end of the oesophagus, stomach, duodenum, small and large intestine, rectum and anus. In addition to these are the spleen, kidneys, liver, pancreas and gall bladder, and the contents of the pelvis which include the bladder, urethra and organs of reproduction.

Rupture to any of these can occur as the result of trauma. The degree of damage and the clinical signs will vary in their times of onset, depending on the severity and nature of impact, and on whether the organs are encapsulated like the spleen.

We cannot list every possible injury to the abdomen in this book, but here are some primary features of abdominal injury as an overview:

▶ pain and guarding in the conscious patient
▶ the abdomen when felt by hand is unyielding
▶ distension
▶ shoulder tip pain on lying down (splenic rupture)
▶ haematemesis or rectal bleeding.

Diagnosis
Diagnosis of an intra abdominal injury is usually made on clinical examination. However, where bleeding is suspected but not confirmed, diagnostic peritoneal lavage may be undertaken. This procedure uses the following equipment prepared by the nursing staff:

1. Dressing trolley and suture pack.
2. Appropriate gloves for the medical staff carrying out the procedure.
3. Local anaesthetic (Lignocaine 1%) and a 10ml syringe and green needle to draw up and orange needle to administer the local anaesthetic.
4. Betadine solution for skin prep.

5. A scalpel with blade (size 15).
6. Peritoneal lavage catheter.
7. Normal saline and administration set.
8. Suture (4/0 Ethilon or similar material).
9. Dry gauze dressing and tape.

After local anaesthetic, if the patient is conscious, the skin is prepped and an incision made 2cm below the umbilicus, travelling in a longitudinal direction.

The peritoneal catheter is then fed through to the peritoneal cavity. The giving set has by now been primed with the normal saline solution. It is attached to the peritoneal catheter, and the litre of normal saline (preferably warmed) is run through and the flow regulator locked off.

The empty bag is then lowered to just above the level of the floor and the regulator opened fully to allow the fluid to drain back. Bloodstained fluid may confirm the presence of bleeding, based on which a surgical decision can be taken.

Prior to peritoneal lavage it may be necessary to pass an orogastric tube (nasogastric if no head injury is suspected) which will require aspirating in order to empty the stomach.

If a pelvis X-ray has excluded a pelvic fracture then a urinary catheter may be passed in order to empty the bladder prior to peritoneal lavage.

Pelvic injuries can be potentially fatal. A large volume of blood can be lost from pelvic fractures; viscera and organs such as the bladder and urethra can rupture. At an early stage an anterio-posterior X-ray of the pelvis is taken in the resuscitation room, as part of a series of three films taken of the cervical spine and chest before it.

The bones of the pelvic girdle need to be examined closely both clinically and radiologically. Fractures to the pelvic girdle if unstable need to be externally fixated. This is very often carried out by the orthopaedic surgeons in the resuscitation room with assistance from operating theatre staff. To move a patient with an unstable pelvic fracture could cause bleeding to increase and that could prove fatal.

Never pass a urinary catheter on a patient with a suspected or confirmed pelvic fracture.

Spinal injury

In trauma, spinal injury at any level is significant. The most vulnerable area is the cervical spine because it is the least protected. It is the level at which nerves that control basic functions such as breathing are to be found.

Protection of the cervical spine is provided in three ways:

1. In-line immobilisation with the patient lying on his back.

2. The use of a spinal board with blocks and straps to prevent mobility of the head and body for as long as appropriate to confirm or exclude spinal injury.

3. A correctly sized and fitted semi rigid collar.

In the absence of the latest technology in spinal immobilisation the minimum standard to immobilise a cervical spine is:

▶ collar
▶ sandbags
▶ tape.

X-rays

Portable X-rays are taken in the form of a lateral view of the cervical spine. These are done in the resuscitation room as soon as the immediate life-threatening problems in airway breathing and circulation have been dealt with. In isolation a lateral film will not exclude a cervical spine fracture. Formal films will be required in the X-ray department before releasing the patient from cervical spine immobilisation.

The log roll

The second aspect of spinal management in trauma is the log roll. This procedure is aimed at rolling the patient in one plane to examine the patient's back and do a rectal examination to check for muscle tone. This procedure needs one person to control the head (not a junior nurse) and three to take up positions along the length of the patient's body. The positions on the body are taken up with the tallest at the head and the shortest at the feet.

Hand positions are then taken up as follows:

1. tallest person with one hand over the scapula, the other over the top of the pelvis

2. second tallest places the hand nearest the patient's head end through the arm of the tallest person to place the hand above the

top of the pelvis, and the other hand is placed under the knee joint furthest away

3. the shortest person places both hands under the ankle furthest away.

The person taking the head gives clear instructions on when the patient is to be rolled. While the patient is in the lateral position the examining doctor feels the entire length of the spine and performs a rectal examination.

If clearing the body of clothing and glass debris is practical, then this is done carefully, and the patient rolled back in the same way to a supine position. If any of the log rolling team become tired then it is important to say so, rather than to risk dropping the patient and causing more serious injury.

Peripheral limb injuries

These have been discussed in earlier chapters. However a few serious ones require mention in the context of trauma management.

Most A&E departments in the UK manage trauma through the principles of the advanced trauma life support guidelines. So far we have considered the management of trauma in the context of the 'primary survey'. This is designed quite rightly to focus on life threatening problems and to correct those before moving on to look at injuries in more detail. A top to toe examination forms the 'secondary survey' in which peripheral limb injuries are identified.

The injuries requiring immediate attention – at least on a temporary basis – are those where dislocation, displaced fractures, or compound fractures are suspected. If the patient is unconscious such injuries can be dealt with quite easily through reduction of the dislocations, straightening and splinting displaced fractures, and covering compound fractures with an iodine based dressing.

Any dressings placed onto open wounds in these circumstances should have paraffin gauze nearest the skin, to reduce difficulties in removing the dressing for definitive care. Limbs with obvious fractures can be placed in temporary plaster of Paris back slabs, pending more definitive management.

For conscious patients analgesia is needed to alleviate the pain from the injury and the corrective procedures detailed above. For this reason it is desirable to use an opiate dug such as morphine. The maximum intravenous dose should be 10mg, preceded by Metochlopramide 10mg in adults to counter any feelings of nausea. Alternatives to intravenous analgesia include nerve blocks such as radial or ulna blocks, or femoral blocks for fractures of the femur. There is no truth in the theory that giving analgesia masks symptoms that might be important later on. Trauma patients are in pain and there is no excuse for withholding pain relief.

It is important to preserve the vascular supply to the limb. Injuries that look to compromise this are dealt with as soon as immediate resuscitation has been completed.

Compound wounds require intravenous antibiotics. Tetanus vaccination should also be given if appropriate.

Burns and scalds

A burn is caused by dry heat; a scald by moist heat. Popular terms can become mixed up when we talk of a chemical 'burn'. After all, a chemical solution is moist and should therefore be classed as a scald. For practical purposes in A&E it doesn't matter about the academic terminology.

What does matter is the depth of the burn or scald. There are three depths that are recognised as:

superficial	epithelial layers
partial thickness	epithelial and dermis
full thickness	deep structures involved.

The amount of body surface area occupied by the burn can be calculated using a burns chart. You should be able to find a copy of one in the resuscitation room.

Calculations only apply to partial and full thickness burns. Superficial burns are managed on a basis of pain relief, deroofing or aspiration of blisters, and dressing according to local policy.

The only superficial burns to require the patient's admission are those greater than 10% in body area, or those that surround the circumference of the neck. Admission of children may vary from these guidelines and also be affected by child protection issues.

Burns of larger proportion have to be considered in two contexts:

1. distributive shock
2. function and disfigurement

Shock arises from the inadequate tissue perfusion brought about as a result of plasma being lost to the extracellular spaces and therefore no longer in the general circulation, generating exactly the same symptoms as described in hypovolaemic shock.

The only difference in dealing with burns is that in addition to the blood tests outlined in hypovolaemic shock it is also necessary to measure a haematocrit.

It is important to establish the exact time of the burn. This will be needed to calculate the formula for fluid replacement, which will be human albumin as opposed to blood. Pain relief is sometimes managed with diamorphine rather than morphine.

The nursing role in major injuries

The nursing role in major injuries can be summarised as follows:

1. preparation for the arrival of the patient
2. transfer of the patient to the A&E trolley and cutting clothing for IV access
3. initial and serial observations
4. maintenance of fluid balance
5. provision of drugs
6. assistance with treatments and log rolling
7. escorts and transfer to appropriate care
8. care of property.

Summary

▶ The principles of advanced trauma life support apply to all trauma patients beginning with airway with cervical spine control breathing, circulation, disability and exposure.

▶ Definitive airway through intubation is indicated for unconscious or shocked patients, in order to avoid hypoxia.

▶ Life threatening conditions must be dealt with before other injuries.

Helping you learn

Progress questions
1. Name two symptoms of tension pneumothorax.
2. Name two symptoms that should raise suspicion of an abdominal injury.
3. What fluid would you prepare for a diagnostic peritoneal lavage?

Seminar discussions
1. A patient has been assaulted and the police request his clothing for forensic examination. How do you deal with this request?
2. Through a chance meeting in the corridor, a patient's relative makes it known to you personally that a trauma patient does not wish to receive a blood transfusion on religious grounds. What do you do, and who do you talk to?

Practical assignment
Take a few minutes to study the contents of the resuscitation equipment in your department. Make a list of the things likely to be needed for a trauma patient.

Surgical Emergencies

One-minute summary – The specialities of general surgery – ear, nose and throat, maxillo-facial, ophthalmic and gynaecology – form the surgical workload in A&E before the patient is referred to the appropriate specialist. Not all patients referred to a surgical team will need an operation. After referral from A&E some will be discharged with appropriate follow up. Taking a sequential, logical and accurate history is important in the case of all patients, especially when the diagnosis may lead to very invasive treatment.

In this chapter you will learn about:

▶ general surgical emergencies
▶ maxillo-facial surgical emergencies
▶ ear, nose and throat surgical emergencies
▶ ophthalmic surgical emergencies
▶ gynaecological and obstetric emergencies.

General surgical emergencies

Abdominal pain

A junior nurse is not expected to diagnose a patient presenting with abdominal pain. However, the junior nurse should recognise the symptoms typical of conditions that require urgent attention. These symptoms are:

▶ pain is severe and of sudden onset
▶ patient vomits repeatedly
▶ patient looks pale and generally unwell
▶ patient vomits blood or passes blood from the rectum
▶ patient's skin colour is altered, suggesting a jaundiced appearance
▶ abdominal pain associated with pregnancy.

Acute surgical conditions that can present as abdominal pain include:

▶ Appendicitis, cholecystitis, peptic ulcer perforation, intestinal obstruction, pancreatitis and peritonitis.

▶ Conditions affecting the rectum and genitalia in A&E are mainly confined to acute abscess formation in the perianal or ischiorectal areas, and torsion of the testicle in the male. Both conditions require a recorded temperature and a surgical opinion.

Two conditions are worthy of special attention – dissecting aortic aneurysm, and renal colic.

Dissecting aortic aneurysm

This is a rupture to the walls of the aorta. It is due to a weakness that causes widening resulting in bleeding through the layers of the vessel. The cause is unknown. The symptoms depend on the level of the aorta affected. Thoracic or abdominal aneurysms can present with a distension and pulsating area over the umbilicus of the abdomen, coupled with pain radiating to the back.

As hypovolaemic shock occurs the patient feels dizzy and looks pale, with all the signs of shock described in the chapter on trauma. The pulses on both sides may be unequal in volume or presence, if the aneurysm is above that level.

This is an extreme emergency requiring immediate attention. Occasionally an ultrasound scan may be performed if the patient is reasonably well and the diagnosis uncertain. A decision to perform surgery can be difficult if the patient is a poor anaesthetic risk.

Renal colic

Loin pain, nausea, vomiting and haematuria are the main symptoms of renal colic. The condition arises due to calculus or stones forming in the renal tract. The site for these stones is usually in the ureters. The blood seen in the urine is due to mild trauma to the ureter as the stone pushes through it.

As considerable spasm is involved in renal colic, it is reasonable to give a drug that will act on smooth muscle, as well as administering conventional analgesia. For this purpose a drug such as Hyocine (Buscopan) 20mg per ml is given by intramuscular injection at a dose of 10 to 20mg or Voltarol (Diclofenac) injection 75mg given intramuscularly as a 3ml injection.

If admission is considered to be appropriate then it is normally arranged under the care of the urologists. A sample of urine should be taken, tested for Leucocytes Nitrites blood and protein, and sent to the laboratory for red cell count and culture and sensitivity in these patients.

Sadly, the symptoms of renal colic become the choice of some individuals to sustain their opiate dependence with elaborate and convincing histories and devious methods of providing a urine sample to show blood on testing. While it is desirable that such individuals are exposed and denied the opiates that they seek, it would be far worse to deny analgesia to somebody in genuine need. So accept such patients at face value and leave the detective work to more senior staff.

Head injury
Uncomplicated head injuries
If the patient has not been knocked out, and shows only transient dizziness and nausea without the presence of a skull fracture, then it is reasonable for the patient to be discharged with a head injury advice card.

This card details the symptoms to be looked out for over the next 48 hours. The patient should return if he/she or their relatives are worried. It is important to give the head injury card to the person accompanying the patient. Patients should have some form of adult supervision when leaving hospital after a head injury.

Scalp wounds
In the absence of a fracture, scalp wounds can be managed in the same way as any other wound. There is the option to close the wound with wound glue or sutures. Adhesive strips are not recommended for scalps because of poor adhesion due to hair. Inspection under a good light, removal of foreign bodies, and irrigation, should be carried out prior to wound closure. Hair ties can also be used.

Bleeding from scalp wounds can be severe with systemic effects of mild hypovolaemia in some cases. If you see profuse bleeding from a scalp wound then tell a more senior nurse; it may be necessary to place some deep holding sutures in the wound if the vessel that is bleeding is not obvious to the naked eye.

Skull fractures
Closed linear fractures without neurological signs will heal without

complication in most cases. However, admission is often indicated as a precaution. Considerable force is needed to produce a skull fracture, so overnight observation is a perfectly reasonable step. Fractures that are comminuted, depressed, or compound need neurosurgical intervention. This is because complications can arise from pressure caused by a depressed segment, and there is potential for a meningeal infection from a compound injury.

Brain injury
At a junior level it is not necessary to be know every variation of brain injury. The aim of A&E is to make an initial diagnosis and provide immediate care. There are two vital points to remember about significant head injuries:

1. The primary symptom of a significant head injury is a fall or fluctuation in the patient's level of consciousness.

2. A head injury is significant when the patient's level of consciousness fails to improve.

Diagnosis of brain injury in most cases will be through a CAT scan. CAT stands for computerised axial tomography. A general anaesthetic is necessary in most cases. Escorting a patient with brain injury should never be the job of a junior nurse.

Maxillo-facial surgical emergencies

Facial fractures
The facial skeleton is complex, both in terms of bony structure and the compressible spaces that form the sinuses. In trauma and severe infection these spaces can fill with fluid and blood. The fluid then creates potential airway problems, infection, and dysfunction to surrounding organs.

Here are seven points to bear in mind when dealing with facial fractures:

1. Trauma is direct, and results from common causes such as assault, fall and road traffic accident.

2. Head injury should always be considered first in patients showing facial injury.

3. Disturbance in vision, taste and smell can arise from compression on branches of the oculomotor, dental, facial, olfactory and lingual nerves.

4. Fractures are classified according to the 'Le Fort' method of lower, middle and upper third fractures being termed 'Le Fort 1, 2 and 3' respectively.

5. Patients can exanguinate from facial fractures due to the healthy blood supply that the facial skeleton requires.

6. All wounds should be covered before definitive management, and before neurological observations are noted.

7. Infection is a real danger in facial fractures. Antibiotics are prescribed for most patients in the acute stages of injury.

Fractures take on the classification of any other fracture and the chapter on fractures clarifies the detail of this.

Dental pain

Generally this is a problem which presents to A&E in the small hours of the morning or at weekends. Dental pain is only ever managed definitively by a dental surgeon.

The patient presents to A&E because of pain and insomnia. This is either due to an acute problem such as abscess formation, or loss of teeth through trauma, or a complication of recent dental surgery.

In adults the prospects of saving a tooth avulsed through trauma largely depends upon how much time has elapsed between avulsion and reimplantation. For this reason the medical staff will try to replace the tooth after irrigating the socket with saline and return the patient to their dentist for further management.

The avulsed tooth should be handled carefully by the crown, and not the root. This is to avoid damage to periodontal structures.

It is important to establish the whereabouts of the missing fragments or whole tooth, and to rule out the possibility of a fragment being lodged in the soft tissues, or having been inhaled.

Pain arising from infection or other sources requires the services of a dental surgeon sooner rather than later. It is not unreasonable to have the patient ring the dental surgery to establish what the 'on call' arrangements are, even in the small hours of the morning. If the patient is unable to see a dental surgeon then the holding measure of pain relief is required. This is usually through the supply of an oral opiate such

Dihydrocodene or Co-Codamol which can be given in tandem with a non-steroidal anti-inflammatory drug so long as there are no contra-indications such as asthma or a history of peptic ulceration. Patients taking opiates should not drive, operate machinery or take alcohol while on such medication. The British Dental Association has expressed concern around the use of Antibiotics by general medical staff in cases of dental infection although some practitioners may still feel it appropriate to provide antibiotics for the patient.

It should be emphasised that these are merely holding measures. The patient should see a dental surgeon at the earliest opportunity for definitive care.

Bleeding tooth socket
A bleeding tooth socket sometimes arises from trauma, but the vast majority of cases are secondary to dental extraction. The haemorrhage is secondary or reactionary and usually involves back teeth.

These patients require general observations of temperature, pulse and blood pressure. A clear history is also needed to establish whether or not they are on anticoagulant therapy, aspirin, or non-steroidal anti-inflammatory drugs that would affect the clotting mechanism.

In addition to feeling agitated the patient may also feel sick having ingested blood. However, it is saliva more than blood that tends to be lost. Direct pressure through biting on a saline-soaked gauze swab for at least 20 minutes may be enough to stop the bleeding and let the patient go home. The patient should be advised to avoid hot food and drink for the next day or so to prevent vasodilatation and re-bleeding.

If this simple measure fails then the bleeding may be arterial. The on-call maxillofacial surgeon may need to suture the socket in order to stop the bleeding. This is a dental procedure that casualty officers or experienced nursing staff should not attempt.

If the patient is on anticoagulant therapy then a blood sample should be taken for an INR. Referral to the general physicians may be necessary.

Ear, nose and throat surgical emergencies

Problems with the ear that present to A&E are mainly confined to:

▶ otitis, externa and media

▶ retained foreign body
▶ perforation of the ear drum
▶ acute episodes of labyrinthitis
▶ Ménière's disease.

Otitis

Otitis, or inflammation of the auditory canal, should not be presenting to A&E unless the patient is so systemically unwell as to require resuscitative measures. In this case the otitis may merely be the focus for general systemic symptoms that need intervention beyond the confines of ENT.

For those patients who do present, then antibiotics by mouth and/or by ear drops can be prescribed, and the patient referred back to the GP. Purulent discharges from the ear should however be considered significant and may warrant an ENT opinion.

One form of otitis that does require urgent ENT referral is that in which the patient with chronic otitis notices a sudden onset of pain followed by a reduction in discharge. This may be symptomatic of a cerebral problem requiring urgent attention.

Symptoms such as hearing loss or difficulties in balance should be referred directly to ENT. A temperature and blood pressure should be taken on patients with significant symptoms. The blood pressure should be taken with the patient lying and standing to exclude cardiovascular causes of vertigo.

Retained foreign bodies

▶ Impacted ear wax can often produce symptoms of pain and discharge. However, the removal of ear wax is a procedure reserved for the practice nurse in the GP's surgery and not the A&E department.

▶ Foreign bodies if seen can be removed by experienced staff. Most foreign bodies are in practice removed by medical staff.

▶ Insects that enter the ear and remain alive should be removed quickly due to the highly unpleasant symptoms that accompany such a situation.

Perforation of the eardrum

This is caused either by direct trauma such as penetration with a cotton

bud or by indirect trauma in patients who have been close to an area of loud explosion. It can also happen in severe otitis media.
The patient with indirect trauma may well have other more urgent injuries before dealing with the eardrum perforation. However, the eardrum should be inspected and a decision made as to whether conservative or surgical repair is required in addition to antibiotics.

Labyrinthitis and Ménière's disease

Both these diseases present with symptoms of nausea, vomiting, and vertigo. In many cases these patients look pale, tired and 'washed out'. In severe cases general illness results from failure to eat or drink adequately. It is often difficult to perform even simple manoeuvres, such as raising the head from a lying position. In A&E an anti emetic such as Metochlopramide 10mg IV may be helpful but the only definitive care will come from admission to an ENT ward for further management.

Problems relating to the nose

These include:

▶ epistaxis
▶ foreign body retention
▶ trauma
▶ acute sinusitis.

Epistaxis

This is the term used to describe bleeding from the nose. It can occur spontaneously or secondary to trauma. When spontaneous it will be unilateral or bilateral. It is typically the result of excessive nose blowing following a head cold, nose picking (especially in children) and hypertension mainly in the elderly.

In many cases, one quite simple first-aid measure will work if properly applied. Sit the patient well forward while pinching the bridge of the nose, and asking the patient to breathe through the mouth for at least 20 minutes. If some ice can be wrapped in gauze to apply over the bridge of the nose at the same time, then so much the better. The procedure should then enable the patient to go home, with advice to rest for the next 24 hours and avoid hot fluids or hot food so that vasodilatation will not arise to cause the bleeding to start again.

More severe nose bleeding will give rise to symptoms of the patient experiencing clots running to the back of the throat and nausea due to swallowed blood. The patient is also very agitated and anxious. This sort of bleeding normally comes from the postnasal area, which is the province of an ENT specialist.

For nose bleeds that continue despite the measures taken above it will be necessary to pack the nose. In most departments this will mean referral to ENT. Some departments not blessed with an ENT service on site may resort to silastic packs or wicks designed to remain in position for 24 to 48 hours.

The recording of blood pressure, pulse and respiratory rate is important for these patients. For them, the danger of hypovolaemia should not be under estimated. Patients on anticoagulant therapy or aspirin are at particular risk. A patient with a nosebleed who is systemically unwell requires full resuscitation protocols and immediate ENT input.

Foreign bodies in the nose are more common in children than adults and their ease of removal will depend upon how visible and accessible they are and how solid they are. With good patient cooperation, most objects can be removed with a pair of Tilleys forceps, local anaesthetic spray and a good light source. Removal of the object will usually be all that is required to resolve the situation, whereupon the patient can go home.

Trauma to the nose

Trauma to the nose will produce bleeding, soft tissue swelling or fractures. Two problems are important to bear in mind when dealing with trauma to the nose:

(a) Trauma to the nose automatically implies a potential head injury until proved otherwise.
(b) A septal haemotoma, which is visible on clinical examination, requires ENT admission for decompression.

Fractures to the nose produce a lot of swelling and deformity, but unless there are immediate airway problems there is no value in X-raying the nose at the time of injury. In 5 to 10 days the patient is seen in the ENT outpatients department. A decision will then be made as to whether the deformity is functionally and cosmetically acceptable or whether a surgical correction is indicated.

Sinusitis

Sinusitis is the inflammation of the air spaces that lie in the facial bones and that are lined with mucous membrane. Infection is the usual mode of inflammation that results in fluid gathering in the sinus that causes pressure and discomfort over the cheek and face with a nasal discharge in more severe cases.

Headache is usually throbbing in nature and symptoms tend to be worse in the morning. Leaning forward is very painful. The urgency of this condition arises from the potential for more serious cases to require surgical intervention in order to drain the fluid and to investigate other sources of infection such as a chest infection.

The throat

Acute problems involving the throat include:

▶ foreign body obstruction
▶ epiglottitis
▶ peritonsillar abscess (quinsy)
▶ post operative tonsillectomy bleeding
▶ trauma.

Foreign body obstruction is quite common, particularly in adults where small animal bones become lodged in the throat, or in children where small objects, mostly coins, become accidentally ingested.

Two situations arise from foreign bodies to the throat. Either a foreign body genuinely is in situ, or the foreign body has moved further down in normal digestion and has caused a scratch to the throat on its way. In either case any visual inspection of the throat is best left to more experienced staff. No attempt whatsoever should be made to inspect the throat of a child.

An X-ray to demonstrate a lateral view of the neck may be requested. If an object is seen then the patient will be referred to an ENT surgeon for its removal, unless it is superficial enough to be safely removed in A&E.

Foreign bodies to the throat that give rise to the symptoms of stridor require immediate transfer to resuscitation facilities and senior staff to manage the situation.

Epiglottitis is an infection normally caused by Haemophyllis B and which mainly, but not exclusively, affects children. As the epiglottis becomes more inflamed the passage through which air flows becomes narrower, resulting in one of the primary symptoms of stridor on inspiration.

In addition to stridor the patient looks pale and will feel hot due to pyrexia. There will also be evidence of dribbling as swallowing becomes more difficult. This condition is so dangerous because spasm can occur around the epiglottis, causing a complete airway occlusion. The provision of a surgical airway is then the only method of oxygenating the patient. The condition is even more dangerous in children, because airway oedema occurs in a child much more quickly than in the adult.

As a junior nurse you need to seek immediate senior help if this condition presents to you. The main aim is to keep the patient sitting upright, with an unobtrusive source of high flow oxygen gently supplied. This should be maintained until sufficient senior anaesthetic and ENT staff are there. They will confirm the diagnosis and take the patient to theatre for intubation in a safe and controlled environment, followed by intravenous Chlorumphenicol to treat the infection at source.

Under no circumstances should anybody attempt to open the mouth or look at the throat in A&E because this may induce spasm and airway occlusion. Observations should be left for senior staff to deal with when appropriate back up is present. It is essential to offer reassurance to parents and enlist their operation in keeping the child calm and comfortable in the resuscitation room.

Peritonsillar abscess (quinsy)

Peritonsillar abscess, or quinsy, is an infection that arises around the tonsils. It generates the symptoms of pyrexia, sore throat, difficulty swallowing and dribbling of saliva around the mouth. Abscess formation creates pain and immense discomfort along with a feeling of general malaise. Intravenous antibiotics are indicated as soon as possible followed by admission to an ENT ward for possible surgical intervention.

Post operative tonsillectomy bleeding can present as secondary or reactionary haemorrhage. The history will usually be quite straight forward, in that surgery was uneventful and bleeding started spontaneously.

The patient may have a post operative infection demonstrable through a pyrexia, although this is not always the case.

General baseline observations should be taken. Bear in mind that these patients can be clinically shocked such that they warrant further surgery to stop the bleeding. A&E care consists of haemodynamic resuscitation and referral to ENT.

Trauma to the throat
Trauma to the throat can be caused through attempted hanging, asphyxiation or penetrating injury whether by accident or intent. Symptoms will depend upon the nature of the trauma, the level at which the injury is sustained and the effects of bleeding or airway oedema. Any injury that exposes underlying structures needs formal surgical exploration.

Ophthalmic surgical emergencies

Eye problems presenting to A&E fall broadly into three categories:

▶ foreign body and chemical retention
▶ penetrating injuries
▶ disease processes of the eye

Foreign body and chemical retention
Foreign bodies in the eye account for most ophthalmic presentations to A&E. The vast majority are successfully removed without any problem. It is important to take a history including the time that the foreign body entered the eye, and the activity that was being done at the time. An X-ray may be requested for patients who give a history of drilling or grinding, so that the presence of an inter-ocular foreign body can be excluded as a possibility.

Measuring visual acuity
All patients with eye problems require their visual acuity to be measured. This is done by asking the patient to cover the good eye and to read the letters on a Snellen chart. Each line has a number below it that denotes the size of the letters.

The size of letters begins with the largest at 60 descending through 36, 24, 18, 12, 9, 6 and 5. Someone who can read as far down as the 9 line with the right eye and the 6 line with the left is documented as having a visual acuity of R6/9 L6/6. If spectacles are normally worn then they should be left on during the test.

If a patient reads only some of the letters on a line then the vision can be documented as that line minus the missing letters from the same line. For example: 6/9-2.

Staining to detect scratches

As with the throat, a foreign body can be present in the eye or it can create a scratch giving the patient symptoms of a foreign body. It is normal practice to stain the eye with Fluorescein if no foreign body has been detected.

This orange dye will stain green on the surface of the eye if any scratch is detected. Abrasions to the coloured part of the eye known as the cornea are treated with oral analgesia for pain relief and topical antibiotics in the event of an infection developing. The use of antibiotics for preventative treatment in corneal abrasion is strictly speaking out of product licence. Chlorumphenicol is the most common of these. It may be necessary to provide local anaesthetic drops to the eye in order to remove foreign bodies without undue pain.

If this is done then Benoxonate or Amethocaine are two of the most commonly used drops. At least 20 minutes should be given before the patient is allowed home after anaesthetic eye drops. This is because the patient will have no feeling in the eye, and may not be aware should another foreign body enter it. Patching of the eye after local anaesthetic is not commonly practiced now.

Chemicals in the eye

Chemicals pose a rather different problem. Burning and corrosion can destroy tissue within the eye unless the chemical is neutralised and removed. Again, an accurate history is important, including attempts to obtain any data sheets available.

The use of a second chemical to neutralise the first is not generally accepted as good practice. Most chemicals respond to thorough irrigation with normal saline. The technique of eye irrigation is best learned by practical demonstration rather than out of a book.

Penetrating injuries to the eye

Penetrating injuries, as the term suggests, describes those where the penetration of an object could disrupt structures in the eye such as nerve branches, blood vessels, muscle and vitreous fluid.

Such disruption can produce dysfunction or loss of vision. Detachment of the retina, and lacerations involving the conjunctiva, are among the injuries that require very urgent input from an ophthalmic surgeon. As a junior nurse, you are advised not to try removing any penetrating object but rather to seek senior help very quickly and learn from what you see.

Disease processes of the eye

Disease processes of the eye present in several forms to A&E. The most common are welding flash, acute closed angle glaucoma, and conditions arising from the red or painful eye.

Welding flash

Welding flash or 'arc eye' results from ciliary muscle spasm in response to rapid pupil constriction when the eye is suddenly exposed to a very bright source of light such as that of a welding torch.

This condition often presents in the early hours of the morning with the patient in pain and displaying a feeling of irritation, lacrimation, and intense fear of light (photophobia). Symptoms typically begin some hours after exposure. The patient may have gone to bed, but been awoken up by the symptoms, which are intense and very painful.

Treatment at source consists of installing eye drops such as Cyclopentolate. These will release the spasm by dilating, and hence resting, the pupil. However, before doing this, some anaesthetic drops should be applied as outlined above.

Some simple oral analgesia such as Paracetamol may also be reasonable, given that many patients experience headaches with this very uncomfortable condition. If possible, patients should be placed in a darkened room while awaiting treatment. If the wait is likely to be long then have an experienced nurse see the patient and arrange some anaesthetic drops as an interim measure.

Acute closed angle glaucoma

This is an ophthalmic emergency.

In this condition the intraocular pressure exceeds that which can be tolerated by the tissues of the optic nerve head. This results in loss of peripheral vision as well as profound systemic symptoms of hypertension, vomiting and headache. Diabetic patients are particularly prone to this disease.

The disease is treated by diuretics, corticosteroids and eye drops to lower the intraocular pressure and to preserve as much vision as possible.

Patients should be nursed on a trolley and given a high priority in the system.

Red eye

In terms of disease, we can include uviitis and iritis among the group of problems presenting as 'red eye' or 'painful eye'. Conjunctivitis sometimes presents to A&E and is rather unwelcome due to the contagious nature of the condition.

Lacrimation, redness and photophobia characterise the symptoms of this condition. It is treated with Chlorumphenicol and referred if repeated episodes fail to respond to treatment or if there is a purulent discharge from the eye. Conjunctivitis in babies that are newborn require further investigation to exclude a chlamydia infection.

Gynaecological and obstetric surgical emergencies

The most common gynaecological presentations to A&E are:

▶ ruptured ectopic pregnancy
▶ threatened and spontaneous abortion
▶ retained foreign body
▶ urinary tract infection.

Ruptured ectopic pregnancy

This is by far the most life threatening gynaecological emergency that will present to A&E. Basically, pregnancy exists but the foetus has developed in the fallopian tube; this has created pressure, then rupture, as growth of the foetus reaches a crucial stage at around 12 weeks' gestation. Symptoms begin with one-sided pelvic pain leading to dizziness, especially on standing, and all the signs of hypovolaemic shock (which may not be accompanied by vaginal bleeding).

Management of this life threatening condition is exactly the same as for any patient in hypovolaemic shock. The definitive management lies in the transfer of the patient to theatre for emergency surgery.

Spontaneous abortion

Spontaneous abortion affects about 30% of pregnancies. There is an increased risk in women over 35, diabetics, and those with thyroid disease. Symptoms usually begin with cramps to the lower abdomen and vaginal bleeding which takes the form of clots. If the foetus is not passed completely then surgery is necessary to prepare the uterus for future pregnancy.

These patients require analgesia, referral and admission for definitive care. The psychological trauma suffered by women who experience spontaneous abortion can be enormous. Although the acute presentation in A&E is not the place for elective psychological care, there is much to be said for taking the time to listen and to provide as much psychological care as is practical.

Retained foreign body in the vagina is a common presentation, due normally to tampon retention. A temperature should always be recorded in these patients because toxic shock syndrome begins with pyrexia. All patients with pyrexia need to be evaluated carefully. Removal of the tampon should be carried out by a doctor or nurse with appropriate experience.

Other foreign bodies are managed in the same way. However, much depends upon the nature of the substance retained. Degradable substances, for example, require surgical removal.

Urinary tract infection

This is far more common in the female than the male because the female urethra is shorter. Many episodes of urinary tract infection present as abdominal pain. In such patients a temperature should be recorded, a urine sample taken for testing, and a pregnancy test carried out. Antibiotics will be provided in most cases.

Pregnancy testing should be carried out with the patient's knowledge and consent except where the patient is unconscious as in trauma.

Summary

▶ Surgical specialities cover a wide range of areas including neurosurgery, ENT, gynaecology, maxillo-facial and general surgery.

▶ A sequential and logical history is important if an accurate diagnosis is to be made and invasive procedures carried out.

▶ Special attention should be given to observing for signs of hypovolaemic shock.

Helping you learn

Progress questions

1. Name the areas of the face that correspond to the Le Fort classifications 1, 2 and 3.

2. Give two symptoms consistent with an aortic aneurysm.

3. What observations would you perform on a patient with a bleeding tooth socket?

Seminar discussion

A patient with an aortic aneurysm is in hypovolaemic shock and needs to be taken to theatre immediately but he is too ill to sign a consent form. How should the medical staff deal with the issue of consent in these circumstances?

Practical assignments

1. Ask a senior colleague to teach you how to do a pregnancy test.

2. Find a Snellen Chart and learn how to assess visual acuity.

Paediatric Emergencies

One-minute summary – The age definitions for a neonate, infant and child are: up to one month, one year, and sixteen years old respectively. The term 'adolescent' is not recognised because it is open to too much interpretation. Some local authorities will keep a child on the 'child protection' register until their seventeenth birthday. Recognition of the sick child is a key part of the knowledge base required by a junior nurse in A&E. Learning how to calculate the weight of a child, and where to look to establish the correct drug dosage, are other vital skills.

In this chapter you will learn:

▶ how to recognise a sick child
▶ common clinical emergencies
▶ your role in child protection
▶ the Children Act
▶ sudden infant death.

Recognising a sick child

As with many situations in A&E it is not for a nurse at a junior level to reach a firm diagnosis in a patient who presents looking unwell. However, that nurse should be able to identify when a patient is sick so that senior staff can be contacted quickly.

The sick child
The two modes by which a child becomes sick are:

1. respiratory failure
2. shock.

However, children have far greater compensation periods than adults. During clinical observations, blood pressure for example may appear quite normal. However, when compensatory mechanisms fail the deterioration in a child is rapid. A cardiac or respiratory arrest in a child is a desperate situation.

Signs of sickness in a child

The indications that a child is sick are:

▶ reduced level of consciousness and failure to recognise parents

▶ rapid respiration with increased labour leading to sternal recession

▶ the child looks pale and capillary refill time is greater than 2 seconds

▶ flaring around the nostrils, indicating an effort to increase the volume of oxygen intake

Be alert to histories that involve convulsion, loss of consciousness, failure to take fluids or pass urine, or where there is evidence of a high temperature or rash. These need to be managed urgently, and you should make senior staff aware of such situations promptly.

The importance of listening and acting on the observations of parents cannot be over-emphasised. Parents know their children. The voiced concerns of parents are usually well founded.

The resuscitation of children

The resuscitation of children is a very stressful process. You will need very clear guidance from experienced staff in the resuscitation room. Children in cardiac or respiratory arrest need to be managed using a logical team-based approach.

This approach will follow Resuscitation Council (UK) guidelines, along with the systems of care published in the Paediatric Advanced Life Support (PALS) and APLS manuals. Copies of these manuals are held by the doctors and nurses who have completed those respective courses.

The principles of resuscitation that you should have some knowledge of are:

▶ Oropharyngeal airways begin at size 000 and move through sizes 00, 0, 1, 2, 3, and 4. They are measured in the same way as for adults (see medical emergencies) but in babies the airway should not be inserted upside down because of the risk of damaging the developing hard palate.

▶ Suction apparatus needs to be adjusted so that paediatric yankeur suckers and catheters are attached to the connecting tubing. The suction power on the unit must be altered from the maximum setting to one that senior staff judge appropriate for the child.

▶ Oxygen needs to be driven at 10 to 12 litres per minute. The non rebreathing mask, or bag valve mask device, should be of the paediatric as opposed to the adult variety. The same applies to any anaesthetic circuit, or defibrillation paddles set up by more experienced staff.

▶ The weight of a child will determine all drug and infusion regimes. The formula for calculating prescriptions is based on an average birth weight of 3.5kg, doubled at six months and trebled at nine months. From age one year the child's weight can be estimated using this formula:

$$(age \times 2) + 8.$$

▶ Where possible a child should be weighed accurately.

▶ Intravenous access can be difficult in children. The type of cannula used will vary according to the preference in your department. You need to make yourself familiar with the various types of cannula so that you can make them available when required. If intravenous access fails in children under six years, intraosseous cannulation will be attempted. The detail of this procedure is outside the scope of this publication.

▶ A fluid challenge is administered during resuscitation. This usually consists of a crystalloid solution such as Hartmans. In some cases a solution such as human albumen may be used. Either way the fluid is administered via a syringe as a bolus at 20mg per kg. Such a challenge may be repeated during the resuscitation.

▶ The size of an endotracheal tube for a child is based on this calculation:

$$\frac{age\ in\ years}{4} + 4$$

▶ You may be asked to help move an intubated child. Great care is needed for this, because endotracheal tubes of size 6 and under are not cuffed. They are secured only by the tape around the mouth. A tube can easily slip causing airway compromise and hypoxia.

▶ All drugs administered to children need to have the dose calculated according to the child's weight. The child's weight should be measured on an accurate set of scales. This is better than using the weight estimation method stated above, but may not be possible in life threatening situations. Some departments use a Broslow tape. When placed along the length of the child this indicates dosages for common drugs and fluid regimes.

▶ As well as recording baseline observations in sick children, a capillary refill time should always be recorded. The size of cuff used in blood pressure measurement should be appropriate for the size of the child. Pulse oxymetry needs to be established using a paediatric probe.

▶ Taking an accurate temperature measurement is necessary in all children in order to exclude pyrexia, which most agree exists at temperatures above 37.4 degrees. Tympanic thermometers provide an accurate, quick and painless means of temperature recording.

Common clinical emergencies

Febrile convulsion
Infection is the usual trigger for the child's core temperature to rise. The temperature regulating centre in the brain becomes affected such that convulsions occur. When the source of infection is treated the temperature will fall. At the time of presentation in A&E the management is focussed on protecting the child's airway, preventing hypoxia and stopping the convulsions.

Your role as a junior nurse in this situation is to summon help immediately and to leave airway management to more senior staff. You may be required to obtain the drugs needed for initial management of the convulsions. These drugs would consist of rectal Paracetamol administered via suppositories. These are stored in the refrigerator along with rectal diazepam, which would be administered if a vein could not be accessed to administer intravenous muscle relaxants.

If muscle relaxants fail to work then paraldehyde is considered. For this gloves must be worn and the solution mixed in arachus oil. The next stage is to use Phenitoin via an infusion pump, which may also mark the point at which intubation is necessary.

Febrile convulsion is a terrifying condition for parents to witness. It is vital that somebody reasonably senior gives them an honest and accurate explanation of what is happening.

Respiratory disease

Asthma, croup, bronchiolitis, epiglottitis and upper respiratory tract infection are the main reasons for presentation to A&E when a child experiences difficulty breathing. Epiglottitis is covered in the chapter on ENT.

As with shock, the point at which a child reaches respiratory failure is always preceded by a stage of compensation where the respiratory function may appear normal or only slightly impaired.

The main task is to identify such children very quickly and begin the interventions that will reverse the path towards respiratory failure. Nebulised Salbutamol is a common first line intervention. Make sure you know how to assemble a nebuliser within your department.

Position of the child

Keeping the child in a position of comfort is important. The conscious child will be most comfortable sitting forward. Have a parent support the nebuliser, at least to start with, remembering to keep the nebuliser upright so that the contents remain in the chamber.

Monitoring

Pulse oxymetry and cardiac monitoring should be available for any child whose respiratory function is causing concern. An escort to X-ray or to the definitive care facility is essential.

Diarrhoea and vomiting

If this is not due to bacterial or viral infection then the cause may be some surgical problem such as intussusception, or a medical problem such as accidental ingestion of a gastric irritant. If symptoms persist, dehydration can lead to hypovolaemic shock, especially in an infant.

The assessment of a child presenting with diarrhoea and vomiting needs to focus on the haemodynamic stability of the patient. Quick action is needed to reverse signs of shock.

Mild cases may be sent home with instructions to maintain fluid intake and move on to normal feeding gradually. A solution that contains electrolytes can often help in the acute stages of illness.

Baseline observations
All children with diarrhoea and vomiting require a full set of baseline observations. These should include:

▶ temperature
▶ pulse (or apex beat in the baby)
▶ blood pressure
▶ respiratory rate
▶ capillary refill
▶ BM reading.

Trauma
The development of bone, organs and soft tissues in children follows broad landmarks at each stage of growth from conception to puberty, at which point the process of ageing is said to begin.

In the context of trauma recognition, management of the sick child is the same as for systemic illness. The principles of trauma management are identical to those outlined in the chapter on trauma.

Child anatomy for trauma
Certain anatomical and developmental differences between adults and children are relevant to trauma. They can be summarised as follows:

▶ Bones are more flexible in children. Fractures often appear as bends or buckles in the contour of the bones.

▶ Growth plates exist at the end of long bones. Damage to these can cause problems in development of the bone.

▶ The anterior and posterior fontanels fuse at about 18 months. This will change the appearance of skull X-rays compared to those of an adult.

▶ The airway of a child is narrow compared to that of an adult. If oedema occurs the diameter of the airway will reduce mathematically to the power of 4. This underlines the importance of good clinical observation and airway management in the paediatric patient.

▶ In healthy children the blood supply is plentiful for wound healing. Many wounds that require sutures in an adult can be closed with less invasive materials in the child.

Pain relief for children
Pain relief in children is important. There can be no reason to leave a child with a burn, or obvious fracture, in pain pending investigations or referrals.

Intravenous opiates are the drugs of choice. They should be drawn up, titrated to 5 or 10mls, and given through a cannula that has been well secured and flushed. Intramuscular analgesia is not considered to be an optimal method of treatment.

The use of Oromorph is valid in some cases. It should be administered according to the recommended dosage bearing in mind that this drug comes in several strengths. This drug is administered orally.

Your role in child protection

Your role in non-accidental injury
The investigation of physical, psychological and sexual abuse is the province of social services. As nurses we have a duty to report situations where abuse is suspected. Each health region should have a nurse dedicated to providing advice on matters of child protection. A policy will exist as to the role of A&E staff when dealing with suspected abuse.

The issue of child abuse needs to be seen in proportion. These children form a very small minority of the total paediatric population in A&E. As a junior nurse it is your duty to make any concern known to a senior member of nursing staff. You should seek guidance regarding any documentation or reporting.

Do not commit pen to paper before talking the situation over with a senior colleague. You should never write '?NAI' or other similar 'codes' in patient notes. To do so constitutes a very serious allegation that you may have to account for personally at a later stage.

Signs of possible non-accidental injury
Talk to a senior colleague if you encounter the following signs when dealing with a child in A&E:

▶ delay in presentation after injury
▶ history that is inconsistent with the injury
▶ poor eye contact by the child and failure to relate to parents
▶ evidence of multiple unexplained bruising of different vintages
▶ direct allegations from the child.

Common injuries in child abuse

Three groups of injury are common in child abuse: 1. physical 2. psychological 3. sexual. Be aware of:

▶ a child on the 'child protection' register
▶ tear to the frenulum of the upper lip
▶ spiral fractures in long bones
▶ fractures in children under one year old
▶ scalds to the underside of both feet from allegedly stepping into a bath (the second foot would not go in after the first had experienced pain).

Despite individual feelings, and political opinion, smacking is not illegal in the UK. The line between chastisement and abuse is a fine one. Most agree that to cause a bruise constitutes abuse.

Sexual and psychological abuse presenting in A&E is rare and should only be dealt with by senior medical and nursing staff.

Never confront an adult about suspected abuse. It is not within the competence or experience of a junior nurse to do so. Seek a private place to discuss your concerns with a senior nurse and take guidance from there.

The Children Act

This Act of Parliament was brought onto the statute book with the intention of giving children a greater say in their own decision making. It applies in A&E in one main area:

▶ Children are entitled to consent to their own treatment, or to refuse it, provided that the nurse or doctor with whom they are communicating is satisfied that they are rational and fully understand what they are consenting to or refusing.

Sudden infant death

Few situations in A&E are more harrowing for even the most experienced staff than the death of an infant. It is also by far the most difficult area of bereavement management because of the emotional devastation of the parents. They may well have had an apparently perfectly healthy infant just a few hours ago.

It is important to distinguish between:

▶ the expected death of an infant suffering from a confirmed disease, such as cardiac myopathy

▶ the unexpected death of a previously healthy infant presenting acutely in A&E.

While both are equally tragic, the former will have created some time for preparation and forewarning of death. Support services will almost certainly have been put in place so that those involved have a greater control of and insight about the situation.

A&E obligations in sudden infant death
The professional obligations of A&E nursing staff in the situation of sudden infant death are:

1. To provide the nursing role for what is usually an aggressive resuscitation attempt.

2. To provide accommodation for the parents. This may be within the resuscitation room or in another private location depending on the policy of the department.

3. To assist in a visual examination of the child after resuscitation has been stopped, and to record a temperature to help determine the time of cardiac arrest.

4. To be with the parents when news of the death is conveyed. To provide for their psychological and physical needs from that point until the relatives leave the hospital.

5. To dress the infant so that the parents can hold and cuddle him or her, either in the resuscitation room or in another private area.

6. The option should be given to have a member of the clergy present if it is the wish of the parents.

7. Documentation and labelling prior to escorting the infant to the mortuary.

Official follow up

It is routine for the police to be involved in sudden infant death and to speak with the parents. In most cases this is done with the utmost sensitivity. The police officers, as human beings, will also be affected by the tragedy.

Follow up will depend upon the services and policies of the local area. However, the GP should be informed so that primary health care needs can be met as appropriate. The hospital paediatricians will have been present throughout. They may have follow up procedures of their own.

As a junior nurse you will be taking a 'back seat' in sudden infant death. However it is important for you to learn from the experience for the future. You must feel free to discuss your feelings openly after the event with your mentor or with senior colleagues.

Summary

▶ The age definitions for a neonate, infant and child are: up to one month, one year and sixteen years old respectively.

▶ Recognition of the sick child is an important component of the junior nurse's knowledge base.

▶ The junior nurse should learn how to calculate the weight of a child, and where to look to establish the correct drug dosage. These are vital skills.

▶ The two means by which children become sick are respiratory failure and shock. Remember that children experience much longer periods of compensation than adults.

Helping you learn

Progress questions

1. How much fluid would you draw up as a fluid challenge for a child weighing 20kg?

2. Why do you need to take great care when moving a child with an in situ endotracheal tube that is 6mm or less?

3. What structure can be damaged in long bone fractures of children?

Seminar discussion
A mother does not wish her 15 year old daughter to have her face sutured, despite the child agreeing to the sutures on the advice of the A&E staff. Who is in the right, and why?

Practical assignment
Read the policy for child protection in your department.

Psychiatric Emergencies

One-minute summary – There are three groups of psychiatric illness, known as the neuroses, psychoses and disorders of personality. More recently, deliberate self harm has emerged as a field taken on by liaison psychiatry; this provides a resource for assessment and follow up of those who are medically fit after an overdose or other form of self harm, whether resulting from psychiatric illness or emotional crisis. Neurotic and psychotic disorders differ in that neurotic disorders involve some degree of insight by the patient. Psychotic patients tend to have reduced or absent levels of insight. The patient's admission to hospital, if not voluntary, is secured by using the Mental Health Act 1983. (Currently under review at the time of publication) – act applies to England and Wales.

In this chapter you will gain an overview of:

▶ clinical features of neurotic disorder
▶ clinical features of psychotic disorder
▶ personality disorder
▶ application of the Mental Health Act
▶ dealing with the mentally ill
▶ deliberate self harm
▶ post traumatic stress disorder.

Clinical features of neurotic disorder

The primary feature of a neurotic disorder is that the patient has an insight into their condition. There is usually a traceable cause to trigger the symptoms. The patient often develops disproportionate perceptions about themselves including a sense of self-blame for all that has gone wrong.

Conditions of this type that may present to A&E are:

▶ reactive depression

150

▶ anxiety state
▶ phobic states.

Reactive depression

It is normal for everyone to have times when they feel low. Life generates challenges and situations that make us feel threatened, undervalued, or very pressurised. The difference, however, between this and the clinical features of reactive depression is the degree of symptoms, and the pace of recovery. These last two factors place the patient at considerable physical risk, if left untreated.

The symptoms of reactive depression are:

▶ low mood and self-esteem
▶ repetitive negative slow speech
▶ slow physical movement and poor eye contact
▶ tearfulness with red and sore eyes
▶ early morning wakening
▶ anorexia and weight loss
▶ bowel disturbance (usually through constipation)
▶ increased alcohol and tobacco consumption
▶ anaemia in more severe cases.

The risk of suicidal thoughts developing into serious intention, and then to physical attempts, must not be underestimated in this patient. Two periods produce heightened vulnerability in such a patient:

1. The first comes as the depressive mood lowers, but the patient is still physically capable of attempting self-harm.

2. The second comes when the depressive mood begins to lift. The patient rises from physical exhaustion, regaining physical capability as described earlier.

The patient can also experience depression through other causes without obvious triggers.

Anxiety state

This arises out of an exaggerated mechanism of self-protection. This mechanism produces triggers for worry and anxiety out of proportion to the problem.

Sometimes the anxiety state can be secondary to something else. Examples could be a life crisis that remains unresolved, or behaviour learned from family members or other role models over the years.

Although the symptoms themselves do not endanger the patient's life they are sufficient to be intrusive, and highly distressing for the patient who sees no prospects of recovery ahead. The symptoms of an anxiety state include:

► restlessness, sweating, dry mouth, and palpitations
► rapid urgent speech
► poor concentration or acceptance of reassurance
► tiredness leading to exhaustion
► excessive consumption of tobacco and sometimes of alcohol
► preoccupation with their own fears and problems to the point of obsession.

Phobic states

A phobia is an irrational fear. Phobic states are rare in A&E. They generally develop gradually and are taken care of through the GP. Symptoms arise from exposure to the source of phobia, whether real or imagined. When the source of phobia is removed, the symptoms abate.

Treatment is necessary when the patient takes measures of avoidance so intrusive to their lifestyle that their physical and mental health is put at risk. The symptoms produced through exposure to the source of fear include:

1. palpitations
2. sweating
3. tachycardia
4. feelings of intense fear
5. occasionally a fear of death.

Admission as an in-patient from A&E is rare. Often, some holding measure is sufficient, such as increasing the existing medication, or prescribing a muscle relaxant pending definitive follow up.

Common phobias include:

► arachnophobia   fear of spiders
► agoraphobia   fear of open spaces
► claustrophobia   fear of closed spaces
► hydrophobia   fear of water.

A phobic state is not strictly speaking a psychiatric emergency. Hyperventilation is the usual presenting symptom. This produces carbon dioxide retention because the patient is unwilling to complete the breathing cycle fully and expel air properly.

In severe cases clubbing of the fingers, tingling through the hands, and flexion (tetany) can arise, which only create further distress for the patient.

Rebreathing their own air via a paper (not plastic) bag will correct this situation and return the breathing to normal. Reassurance is everything in this situation. The attention/reward cycle triggered by many of these episodes should be avoided by the nursing staff adopting a kind but firm approach.

Clinical features of psychotic disorder

The fundamental feature of psychotic disorder is a lack of insight by the patient. Patients do not realise that they are unwell. They may have altered perception in their thoughts and experiences that remove them from reality. This is why it is so important for such patients to receive the correct treatment. This may sometimes mean admitting them to hospital against their will.

There are three main conditions that present in this group of disorders:

1. schizophrenia
2. hypomania and manic depressive psychoses
3. hysteria.

Schizophrenia

There are several types of schizophrenia, the most common of which is simple schizophrenia. Others include paranoid, hebephrenic and catatonic. It is beyond the scope of this book to detail the symptoms relevant to each type, but they all have one thing in common – hallucinations.

In schizophrenia the combined symptoms produce a disintegration of the personality, affecting the way the sufferer thinks, feels and behaves. This is not the same as the popular idea of a 'split' personality

A hallucination is an altered sensory perception. Hallucinations can be experienced through all the senses:

▶ visual   through sight
▶ auditory   through hearing (usually voices)
▶ tactile   through touch
▶ gustatory   through taste
▶ olfactory   through smell.

Hallucinations can be accompanied by delusions, which are fixed false beliefs. These delusions can take many forms, for example delusions of grandeur, persecution and poverty.

Once a set of delusions becomes elaborately organised in the patient's mind then a state of paranoia can emerge. For example, patients with delusions of persecution may watch the television news and believe the newscaster is talking about them and plotting to harm them.

The causes of schizophrenia can either be organic or functional. They are organic when a specific physical illness has produced the symptoms. They are said to be functional where the cause is unknown. Among the organic causes are:

1. toxicity
2. cerebral tumours
3. drug and alcohol ingestion/withdrawal
4. diabetes
5. epileptics following a fit
6. hypoxia.

It is for this reason that a full set of observations should be taken – including a temperature and BM reading – before sending the patient for psychiatric assessment.

Hypomania and manic depressive psychoses

Hypomania is a disorder of mood. In days of old, patients were said to be 'manic' when their mood was so uncontrollably high that they would literally be dancing on the hillsides. Nowadays, modern drugs have eliminated the state of mania and have left us with the next stage down, that of hypomania.

The hypomanic patient is susceptible to elevation in mood. This is likely to remain until biochemical influences, and sometimes social triggers, push his mood to the other extreme of manic depression. This second state shows all the signs of reactive depression at its worst, but without any acompanying insight on the part of the sufferer.

On other occasions however the mood may normalise. When the patient is hypomanic the following symptoms can be seen:

▶ Insight is missing – except in more chronic cases. Patients may realise they are 'high' even though they can do nothing to control it.

▶ Flight of ideas – patients are unable to remain sufficiently focused to complete sentences or hold meaningful conversations. Their thoughts are too pressured by a continuous stream of ideas.

▶ Tiredness – patients fail to sleep or eat owing to their preoccupation with the unrealistic schemes that they must complete.

▶ Rapid urgent persuasive speech – used to co-opt those willing to help in grandiose schemes that may at first seem plausible.

▶ Lack of concentration – the patient can be easily led to another subject with minimal cues.

Treatment for these patients actually seems a shame at first, since they live contented with their schemes. However, their distance from reality will soon create problems as the credit card bills drop onto the mat and creditors press for payment. Also, the physical exhaustion resulting from such over-activity will lead to physical illness unless treatment is given.

Sedation in A&E may be given after discussion with the duty psychiatrist. Lithium Carbonate is the drug of choice when considering long term treatment. Blood levels need to be assessed regularly while a patient is taking the drug. Hyperpyrexia and profuse vomiting are two features of Lithium Carbonate overdose, which can be fatal.

Hysteria

The public often think of hysteria as a kind of panic attack. In fact, the condition arises from the over-use of a mental defence mechanism known as displacement.

In broad terms there are three groups of mental defence mechanisms that keep our ego (self) protected:

1. blocking
2. disguising
3. rechannelling.

Displacement is one of the blocking mechanisms.

The word 'hysteria' comes from the Greek term meaning 'wondering uterus'. This implies that the condition is a predominantly female affliction. However a leading example of hysteria was that of soldiers who 'froze' as they came out of the trenches in World War One (1914-18). As they surveyed the horror of what awaited them, many opted out mentally. In effect they underwent a process of psychological removal from the situation, which they were unable to tolerate.

A modern day example of hysteria is the patient who enters A&E, following a traumatic event, with no recall of how he got there or who he is. This is sometimes known as a 'fugue'.

Overview of personality disorder

The term 'personality disorder' is given to people said to have acquired badly learned behaviour, such that they live outside of the normal values and behaviour expected by society.

The common thread running through personality disorders is the regard for 'self', which is above and often at the expense of others. The terms 'psychopath' and 'sociopath' are widely used to describe such people who can be classified according to their traits and intellect.

Many people with personality disorders find their way into an A&E department, prepared to manipulate the system of care. They seek to gain comfort and empathy for themselves with no conscience about the time they take at others' expense or the unreasonable nature of their requests for help. This manipulation can be such that a junior nurse may not recognise it until a very late stage in the patient's stay. The nurse then realises that the tales of woe were in fact a tissue of deception designed to produce the empathy and positive regard that the patient craved.

Many people with personality disorders find their way into the penal system. Other individuals and organisations bring legal cases against them on account of their behaviour. However, these disorders rarely merit admission of the person as a psychiatric emergency. Many of the more severe cases are dealt with electively under the forensic psychiatry services, which do not generally take patients direct from A&E.

Application of the Mental Health Act

The Mental Health Act of 1983 (currently under review) gives appropriate professionals the legal right to detain a patient against his or her will for a set period of assessment and treatment in a psychiatric unit.

A sense of proportion is needed when considering compulsory admission. The vast majority of patients who require psychiatric in-patient care are admitted informally. A few ask to be admitted, but such a request is often declined by the psychiatrist for various reasons.

A very small number of patients are considered to be a danger to themselves or others, and these are the ones admitted under a Section of the Act.

As a junior nurse you have no part to play in the application of a section under the Mental Health Act. The Act will be applied by the medical staff, along with a social worker there to represent the 'layman' and to be an advocate for the patient. The social worker can overturn a decision to admit the patient if they feel that it is not appropriate.

Once the section papers are signed the patient may legally be detained by the use of reasonable force. Where humanly possible negotiation and persuasion should be used to enforce the section. 'Reasonable' force may be used only as a last resort, and by senior experienced staff or the police.

Dealing with the mentally ill in A&E

Even the most experienced nurse finds it difficult to make an accurate assessment of mental illness. As a junior nurse you will just be asked to report what you noted in the patient's physical appearance, heard in his account of events, and any obvious signs that you noticed during the conversation.

Patient aggression

Remember, all patients are human beings with feelings and fears, and aggression is a sign of fear. Most experienced nurses will tell you that physical assaults are made far more often by patients with physical injuries complicated by alcohol, than by patients suffering from a genuine mental illness.

Junior nursing roles for psychiatric emergencies

Here are some general points to bear in mind when dealing with psychiatric emergencies:

1. Always perform baseline observations to rule out physical illness.

2. Do not 'play along' with hallucinations or delusions. It will only serve to reinforce the patient's removal from reality.

3. When dealing with a patient always ensure that a colleague knows where you are. Keep to the outer areas of sealed rooms.

4. Be honest with the patient. Don't make promises that you cannot deliver, because this will only breed a lack of trust later on.

5. Bear in mind that assessments and decisions regarding the most appropriate outcome for a patient can take a very long time.

Overview of deliberate self harm

Once referred to as 'parasuicide', the act of deliberate self-harm can typically take several forms:

▶ drug overdose
▶ self inflicted lacerations
▶ asphyxia through self-hanging
▶ jumping from a height.

Three questions to ask

There are three questions that the nurse should ask regarding any patient who presents following self-harm:

1. Is the patient physically fit to wait?

2. Is the patient prepared to wait given that they may wait quite a while to see a psychiatrist or other appropriate healthcare professional?

3. Is the patient distressed?

If the patient is physically unwell, distressed or not prepared to wait, then a priority should be given above less seriously injured patients. But what legal powers exist to hold a patient in the department, if they show their intention to leave before being seen by a doctor? This is an area of confusion for nurses, yet the legal position is quite clear.

'A danger to himself or others'

You may decide that having witnessed the patient's behaviour he is a danger to himself, or to others. Then, even as a junior nurse, you personally have the common law right to hold the patient, using 'reasonable force' if necessary. In practice that holding power would only apply until a more senior nurse or doctor arrived to relieve you of the situation.

No judge in a court of law will rule against you on this basis providing that you can demonstrate that the patient was a danger to himself or to others, through the actions and symptoms that you personally saw, or through the conversation that you personally witnessed or had yourself with the patient.

You should tell the patient that you are using such powers to detain him pending a more senior assessment. You are acting in the best interests of the patient.

Most patients respond to verbal persuasion when asked to stay in A&E for a completed assessment. Senior staff should be on hand fairly promptly in such circumstances.

Assessing the risk of suicide

Several assessment tools exist to help determine the level of suicidal risk. While it is beyond the scope of this book to detail them, it is worth mentioning some factors that increase the risk of suicide:

▶ previous attempts at deliberate self-harm.
▶ social isolation and poor support at home.
▶ a suicide note.
▶ evidence of measures having been taken to ensure that the patient would not be found.

If a patient is deemed to be at high risk of suicide then close supervision is important. This can include going into the toilet with the patient and not losing sight of the patient for a moment.

Post traumatic stress disorder

Specific symptoms apply to this disorder. A diagnosis can only be made if those symptoms have been present for over a month.

The disorder arises from an event regarded as outside normal life experience. For this reason such events as divorce or bereavement in normal circumstances do not meet that definition. Given that the event and duration of symptoms are appropriate for a diagnosis other specific symptoms are:

1. intrusive thoughts and recollections occupying 80% of the day
2. flashbacks and re-experiencing of the event
3. outbursts of anger.

It is unusual for a patient to present in A&E with this disorder, without having been already diagnosed elsewhere. A patient is more likely to arrive in A&E having reached a crisis point in his symptoms which makes admission to hospital necessary.

No definitive treatment is possible for this patient in A&E. The symptoms and events that accompany this very distressing condition are too complex to manage there.

Summary

▶ Psychiatric illness is broadly grouped under neurotic disorders, psychotic disorders, and personality disorders.

▶ Insight is lacking or absent in psychotic illness but is usually present in the other two groups.

▶ Deliberate self-harm can result from psychiatric illness or be triggered by an emotional crisis often influenced by social factors.

▶ Hallucination, delusions and paranoia characterise psychotic illness.

▶ Admission to hospital is either voluntary or as a result of senior staff applying a section of the Mental Health Act 1983 (currently under review).

Helping you learn

Progress questions

1. Name four symptoms that would accompany reactive depression.
2. What is meant by the term 'delusion'?
3. Under what law would you as a junior nurse detain a patient whom you had demonstrable reason to think was a danger to himself or others?
4. What component of the personality is generally lacking or deficient in patients with psychopathy?

Seminar discussions

1. A patient who has lacerated her wrist through deliberate self harm tells you that she now regrets her actions and would now like to leave the hospital. What do you do?
2. A patient refuses to go into a room that you have allocated for him. He says he can smell gas released by people who want to kill him. Despite this obvious delusion there is no room available elsewhere in the department. How do you deal with this situation?

Practical assignment

Ask a senior colleague to recall the last patient that they cared for who required psychiatric admission and talk the case through so that you understand the symptoms and their intepretation.

Glossary

Abrasion A wound in which the superficial layer of skin (epidermis) is removed as a result of friction.

Analgesia A reduced sensitivity to pain brought about either by damage to sensory nerves or by administering pain-killing drugs.

Anaphylaxis The secretion of histamine from the tissues in response to a specific antigen. This reaction can produce symptoms that are life threatening.

Aneurysm Weakness in the walls of the vessels in the aorta that can produce rupture which is imminently life threatening. Hypovolaemic shock results from massive blood loss over a short period of time.

Angina Deprivation of oxygen to the coronary arteries, thereby producing chest pain, especially on exertion.

Antibiotic General term for any medication derived from micro organisms designed to kill bacteria that grow to produce infection.

Anticoagulant A substance used to stop blood clotting. Examples of synthetic anticoagulants are drugs such as Heparin and Warfarin.

Apnoea The absence of breathing.

Appendicitis Inflammation of the appendix, usually arising from infection. Surgical removal is the usual treatment for this condition. Left untreated it can lead to abscess formation or gangrene at the site of the appendix.

Artery A blood vessel carrying oxygenated blood away from the heart to the tissues. An exception to this is the pulmonary artery that carries deoxygenated blood.

Asphyxia Deprivation of oxygen to the tissues. It results from mechanical obstruction of the airway or from other causes such as toxic gas or chemicals. Symptoms of asphyxia can also be experienced during anaphylaxis.

Asthma A condition involving the narrowing of the respiratory tract resulting in difficulty in breathing and characterised by wheezing and coughing. The symptoms can range from mild feelings of breathlessness and wheezing to life-threatening symptoms of exhaustion and inadequate oxygenation to the tissues.

Avulsion The term used to describe a portion of tissue or fragment of bone that has become removed from it's point of anchor. Mechanism of 'shearing' is common in this situation.

Biceps An important group of muscles situated in the upper arm and the back of the thigh. They enable flexion and extension to take place at the

161

elbow and the knee, as well as supination of the forearm and external rotation of the lower leg.

Bursar A sac made of fibrous tissue and filled with synovial fluid. It is situated mainly over joints thereby allowing free movement at sites where friction may be problematic.

Cardiac arrest A life threatening situation where the heart muscle fails to pump blood to oxygenate the tissues.

Cardiogenic Pathology from the heart producing a state of shock. Cardiogenic shock can arise in myocardial infarction.

CAT scan An X ray investigation using Computerised Axial Tomography to view anatomical structures in slices or layers. Patients with severe head injuries have a CAT scan to diagnose the presence of blood clots or fluid in the brain.

Catatonic A mental state in which the patient is unable to communicate, though still able to hear and process external stimuli. The patient may adopt a static and passive posture, and remain in such a position for long periods of time.

Catheter A tube that can be passed into an orifice for the purpose of widening the orifice or passing fluid through the orifice. The catheter is usually a flexible tube.

Cerebral Relating to the cerebrum (brain).

Colic A spasm of smooth muscle causing acute severe and often intermittent pain. Most references to colic relate to the abdomen.

Comminuted Term used to describe a fracture where bone is broken into several pieces at the same site.

Contusion A bruise caused by direct or indirect trauma and created as the result of capillary bleeding beneath the skin.

Crepitus The noise and palpable sensation created when two ends of broken bones rub together. Crepitus is a sign of potentially unstable fractures.

Croup An inflammation of the larynx and upper respiratory tract in children between the age of six months and three years. Symptoms include shortness of breath and stridor. This condition can often generate symptoms similar to epiglottitis.

Cuniform One of the tarsal bones in the foot at the same site as the cuboid and novicular bones.

Defibrillation The delivery of a DC electrical shock. It is designed to restore the heart muscle from a fibrillating rhythm, that produces electrical chaos, to an electrical rhythm that will sustain a cardiac output sufficient for adequate tissue perfusion.

Dermis The layer of skin below the epidermis. The epidermis is the top layer of skin.

Distal An anatomical term denoting a point away from the midline, or furthest from a point of reference.

Dorsum Anatomical term denoting the upper side of the hand or foot, the side opposite to the palm of the hand or sole of the foot.

Drug A substance capable of bringing about organic change for diagnosis, prevention or cure of illness or symptoms. The drugs administered may take many forms, depending on the patient's constitution, strength and route of administration.

Dysphagia A term used to describe difficulty in swallowing.

Dyspnoea Shortness of breath. This term should not be confused with apnoea, which describes the absence of breathing.

Emergency A situation requiring immediate or urgent intervention in order to save life, or to prevent a situation from becoming life threatening.

Emetic A substance designed to produce vomiting. An antiemetic is therefore a substance designed to prevent vomiting.

Endoscopy A clinical procedure allowing the upper gastrointestinal tract to be viewed by means of an endoscope. This is a flexible fibre optic tube with a light source capable of being passed through narrow orifices.

Epiglottitis An infection from the haemophilus B bacteria producing swelling and inflammation of the epiglottis. It can occur in adults but is more common, and more acute, in children where airway obstruction can require the provision of a surgical airway.

Epilepsy A condition characterised by convulsions or fits. These may occur either from known causes such as head injury, from febrile states (particularly in children), or through unknown causes.

Epistaxis Term used to describe a nose bleed.

Faciomaxillary The clinical speciality dealing with pathology of the facial skeleton.

Febrile convulsion A fit that occurs due to a high temperature, especially in children.

Gastric lavage A procedure used to empty the stomach. A tube is passed through the mouth and fluid poured into the tube. The fluid is then siphoned out by lowering the tube below the level of the patient.

Geriatric The term used to describe an elderly person in the context of the health care. This term is less fashionable nowadays, with the term 'elderly' normally being preferred.

Glaucoma An ophthalmic emergency where the inter ocular pressure is raised sufficiently to cause blindness. This condition is associated with hypertension and is particularly common among diabetics in their later years.

Gynaecology The clinical speciality dealing with the reproductive system in women.

Haematology The clinical speciality dealing with diseases of the blood.

Haematoma The formation of a blood clot.

Haemoarthrosis A collection of blood in a joint space. It is commonly found at the knee and elbow joints following trauma.

Haemorrhage The loss of blood from the circulation.

Hyperflexion The excessive flexion movement in trauma that occurs at the wrist, fingers, ankle and toes.

Hyperglycaemia A raised blood sugar level. It may lead to the life threatening state of ketoacidosis if left untreated.

Hyperventilation A level of respiratory effort above that required for normal activity. Panic and psychological influences often act as the trigger, but hyperventilation may also arise in cases of metabolic acidosis.

Hypoglycaemia The term used to describe a low blood sugar level. In diabetics this condition can have a rapid onset, and if left untreated can be life threatening.

Hypomania A mood disorder that produces a marked state of excitement and hyper-activity. It is corrected by the use of the drug Lithium Carbonate.

Hypovolaemic Reduction in the volume of circulating blood within the body. A state of hypovolaemic shock will arise when the reduction is such that adequate tissue perfusion is threatened.

Hypoxia The term used to indicate a low level of oxygen in the body. It will produce metabolic and potentially life threatening changes if left untreated.

Infection The transfer of pathogenic organisms between living cells. The transfer can take place in many ways, for example airborne and by droplet infection.

Insulin A protein hormone secreted by the pancreas to control the amount of glucose in the blood stream. Insulin is produced in the form of an injection for patients who are unable to produce sufficient amounts of insulin themselves (diabetic).

Intercostal The area of anatomy between the ribs. Intercostal drainage is the technique of placing a chest drain through this area into the pleural space in order to correct a pneumothorax or haemothorax.

Intubation The insertion of an endotracheal tube through the mouth or nose into the trachea in order to secure a definitive airway.

Ketone A product of metabolism found in diabetic patients who have a raised blood sugar. Ketone is produced as a result of the failure to produce insulin in the pancreas to control the blood sugar. Ketones are detectable in the urine.

Laceration A break in the continuity of the skin produced usually as the result of direct trauma. Lacerations are placed in various classifications.

Lacrimation The production of tears from the eyes from the lacrimal ducts. A failure to produce tears can be the result of damage to the lacrimal apparatus.

Ligament A structure joining two bones at a joint. A ligament is made of fibrous connective tissue.

Log roll The method used to turn a patient in one plane in order to protect the integrity of the spine. This procedure requires four people, as well as the person carrying out procedures such as examination or pressure area care.

Meninges The dura mater, arachnoid mater, and pia mater, that line the surface of the brain to provide protection and accommodation for the circulation of cerebrospinal fluid.

Mentor A fellow professional from whom advice and guidance can be obtained.

Metabolism The process of breaking down food taken into the body into substances the body can use for energy and growth. The process of metabolism also includes the elimination of waste products.

Metatarsal The bones in the foot connecting the large bones of the foot to the toes.

Mucosa Membranes that are lubricated by mucin and other substances designed to protect the surface of the tissues or carry enzymes to other places. The mucus membranes of the mouth are a typical example as saliva is transported to break down the food during mastication.

Myocardial Relating to the myocardium. The myocardium is the middle layer of heart muscle, surrounded by the pericardium and the endocardium. The most common disorder of the myocardium in A&E is myocardial infarction (heart attack).

Nebuliser A device used to administer a drug by inhalation through a mist. The most common drugs are Salbutamol and Iputropium but adrenaline can also be administered in this way.

Neonate A baby in the first four weeks of life.

Neurosis A group of psychiatric disorders characterised by insight agitation and anxiety, phobia, compulsion and obsession.

Neurovascular Term referring to the nerve and blood supply to a given area of the anatomy.

Obstetric The surgical speciality devoted to the management of pregnancy and childbirth.

Olecranon A bony prominence at the elbow.

Olfactory The term used to describe the sense of smell. The olfactory nerve is the third cranial nerve.

Ophthalmic The surgical speciality dealing with pathology to the eyes.

Opiate A drug made with opium as the main ingredient. Such drugs arise from the opium plant and many opiates are classed as controlled drugs. They are primarily used in pain relief, the most common example being morphine.

Organ A group of tissues within the body that form a functional structure.

Otitis Inflammation of the ear. Otitis can occur in the outer ear (otitis externa) or to the middle ear (otitis media).

Paediatric The term used to refer to children. Generally the age of 16 years is regarded as the cut off point into adult medicine.

Palpitations A feeling of rapid heart beat that can produce anxiety and giddiness.

Pancreas A gland situated behind the stomach which secretes insulin and other substances that help the digestion.

Patella The anatomical term for the knee cap.

Pathology The branch of medicine concerned with disease, especially its structure and its functional effects on the body. The term is also used for the speciality which seeks to establish the cause of death.

Peritonitis Inflammation of the peritoneum due to infection. The peritoneum is the lining of the abdominal cavity which is structured in layers.

Phobia An irrational fear that is so intense as to make the patient use avoidance tactics that become intrusive to daily life.

Photophobia A fear of light, often present in patients with meningitis and eye problems.

Pneumothorax The collapse of a portion of lung which can be spontaneous or due to trauma. The pressure in the pleural space moves from negative to positive.

Preceptor A professional colleague who offers guidance in the early portion of one's nursing career.

Pronation The movement of the forearm at the elbow joint in such a way that the palm is facing downwards.

Psychiatry The medical speciality that deals with disease of the mind. This can be organic or functional. All psychiatrists are fully trained medical practitioners.

Psychopath The term used to describe a person who has acquired badly learned ingrained behaviour that is accompanied by lack of social conscience.

Psychosis A group of psychiatric disorders characterised by lack of insight, hallucinations, paranoia and delusion.

Pulse The palpable beat of the heart felt as blood is pumped by the left ventricle into the circulation.

Pulse oxymetry A non invasive machine used to measure the oxygen saturation as a percentage via a sensor that is attached to the ear lobe, finger or toe.

Pyrexia A high temperature. The definition of what constitutes a high temperature is debatable but most agree that a temperature above 37.4 C is raised.

Quadriceps Large group of muscles in the thigh which allow flexion and extension of the thigh.

Quinsy A peritonsillar abscess characterised by marked difficulty swallowing, pyrexia and general malaise. This is an ENT emergency.

Radiology The medical speciality devoted to the collection and interpretation of X rays and scans that detect abnormality within the body.

Reactive depression A clinical depression brought about through a known cause in which the patient retains insight.

Rehydration The process of fluid replacement following dehydration. This can be done through the oral, nasal or intravenous route.

Respiratory arrest The cessation of breathing.

Resuscitation The process of restoring a cardiac and respiratory output sufficient to allow adequate tissue perfusion following trauma or illness.

Sartorius The long muscle in the thigh allowing flexion of the thigh.

Scaphoid Largest of the carpal bones in the wrist and the most common to fracture, although radiological demonstration of this fracture can often be delayed.

Schizophrenia A psychiatric disorder otherwise known as psychosis.

Serous fluid Clear fluid found draining from tissues following injury and infection.

Shock Inadequate tissue perfusion resulting from injury or illness. Primary signs are a pale complexion, rapid pulse, increased respiratory rate and sweating, with low pressure and increased capillary refill time.

Sickle cell anaemia Disease common in populations originating from areas in which malaria is endemic. The oxygen carrying red blood cells take the shape of a sickle which reduces their capacity to transport oxygen to the tissues.

Sociopath Term used to describe an individual who is unable to conform to behaviour expected by mainstream society and who is deemed to be mentally ill as a result.

Spatula A wooden stick rather like the shape and dimensions of a lollipop which is used to flatten the tongue when inspecting the throat or in tightening the traction cord on a Thomas splint.

Spleen An encapsulated organ within the abdomen responsible for the production of red blood cells in the new-born and for the destruction of unwanted cells in the circulation.

Steroid Naturally occurring hormones within the body such as corticosteroids, androgens and oestrogens. Steroids are also synthetically produced and used for the suppression of the inflammatory response in such conditions as asthma.

Stridor The noise produced on inspiration by partial occlusion of the airway. This can occur in situations of epiglottitis or retained foreign body.

Subarachnoid The space under the arachnoid mater that forms part of the meninges that line the brain. Haemorrhage can occur in this area either spontaneously of following trauma.

Subluxation The partial dislocation of a joint.

Supination Movement of the forearm at the elbow joint where the palm is uppermost.

Suture Term used to describe a thread that is used to repair a wound. Also a term used to describe the naturally occurring spaces between the bones of the skull.

Tachycardia A rapid pulse generally accepted as over 100 beats per minute in an adult. Children have different thresholds of tachycardia depending upon their age and stage of development.

Theophylline A group of drugs designed to dilate the bronchus. Used in severe asthma.

Therapy The provision of treatment for the purpose of cure or support in illness or distress.

Thorax The chest cavity incorporating the structures of the lungs and rib cage including the diaphragm.

Thrombolysis The process of providing drugs to break down blood clots in the circulation with particular emphasis on the coronary arteries. These drugs are administered in the early stages of myocardial infarction.

Titration The reconstitution of a drug into a weaker solution than its original concentration. An example would be of titrating morphine from a solution of 10mg per ml to 10mg in 10ml through the addition of 9ml of water or saline.

Toxic Poisonous. Specifically, the term used to describe a state where toxins of a viral or bacterial nature have entered the blood stream to produce symptoms of a raised temperature and malaise. If left untreated can lead to potentially life threatening symptoms of confusion, convulsion and renal failure.

Trachea A cylindrical anatomical structure connecting the upper airway structures to the bronchi.

Trachiostomy A surgical procedure often done as an emergency whereby an opening is created in the trachea to provide an airway, in the event of occlusion in the upper airway.

Trauma An injury or assault to the body. It may be physical, psychological or sexual in nature.

Tremor Uncoordinated shaking usually of the peripheral limbs. It is due to hypothermia, alcohol or drug withdrawal, anxiety or clinical diseases of the nervous system.

Trephine The treatment used to evacuate clotted blood from under a finger or toe nail. The procedure involves burning through the nail to create a hole through which the clot can be released.

Tubigrip The trade name for a product made by Seton. The product is an elastic stocking support for the arms and legs. Other makes of the same product exist on the market.

Ulna The smaller of the two bones in the forearm connecting the elbow to the wrist.

Urea A waste product of digestion found in the bloodstream.

Urethra Anatomical structure consisting of a tube that connects the bladder to the exterior for the passage of urine. The female urethra is short compared to that of the male, making females more prone to urinary tract infections.

Vein A blood vessel carrying deoxygenated blood back to the heart.

Venous Of, or pertaining to, the veins.

Ventricular Referring to the ventricle of either the heart or brain. In the heart, the ventricles are the muscular chambers that pump blood.

Vertigo A condition which affects the sense of balance, producing difficulty in standing and walking, and in many cases nausea and vomiting.

Volar Anatomical reference to the palm side of the hand and forearm, or the sole of the foot.

Further Reading

Acute Care Psychiatry: Diagnosis & Treatment , Lloyd I. Sederer (Editor) & Anthony J. Rothschild (Editor). Hardcover (June 1997). Williams & Wilkins. ISBN: 0683300067
Acute Medicine: A Practical Guide to the Management of Medical Emergencies. David Sprigings, Andrew Jeffrey, John B. Chambers & David Sprigings. Paperback, 448 pages, 2nd edition (August 1995). Blackwell Science Inc. ISBN: 0632036524
Cambridge Textbook of Accident and Emergency Medicine. David Skinner (Editor), Andrew Swain (Editor), Rodney Peyton (Editor), & Colin Robertson (Editor). Hardcover (May 1997). Cambridge University Press. ISBN: 0521433797
Caring for Children. Paperback (1997). BMJ Publishing Group. ISBN: 0727911266
Emergency Management of Skin and Soft Tissue Wounds: An Illustrated Guide. Ernest K. Kaplan, Vincent R. Hentz. Paperback (October 1984). Little Brown & Co. ISBN: 0316482781
Emergency Orthopaedics: The Extremities. Robert R. Simon, Steven J. Koenigsknecht & Robert R. Simon. Paperback, 3rd edition (January 1995). Appleton & Lange. ISBN: 0838522084
Emergency Triage. Manchester Triage Group. Paperback (November 1996)
Management of Major Trauma. (Oxford Handbooks in Emergency Medicine). Colin Robertson & Anthony D. Redmond. Paperback (July 1991). Oxford University Press. ISBN: 0192618245
Minor Injuries and Repairs. John A. Grossman & Sharon Ellis (Illustrator). Hardcover (November 1992). Gower Medical Publishers. ISBN: 1563750805
Paediatric Nursing. Jane Ball & Ruth M. Bindler. Hardcover (August 1994). Appleton & Lange. ISBN: 0838580181
Surgical Emergencies. John R. T. Monson (Editor), Graeme Duthie (Editor) & Kevin O'Malley (Editor). Hardcover (October 1998). Blackwell Science Inc ISBN: 0632050470
Wounds and Lacerations: Emergency Care and Closure. Alexander T. Trott. Hardcover, 416 pages 2nd edition (August 1997). Mosby Year Book. ISBN: 0815188536
Acute Medical Emergencies A Nursing Guide. Richard Harrison & Lynda Daly. Paperback, 404 Pages 46 Illustrations (March 2001). Churchill Livingstone Published. ISBN: 0443064229
Accident and Emergency Theory into Practice. Brian Dolan & Lynda Holt. Paperback 578 Pages 50 Illustrations. Baillière Tindall Published

(November 1999). ISBN: 070202239X

Practical Procedures in the Emergency Department. John Bache. Paperback 176 Pages 297 Illustrations (July 1998). ISBN: 0723430136 . Mosby Wolfe

A Nursing Guide. Richard Harrison & Lynda Daly. Paperback 404 Pages 46 Illustrations (March 2001). Churchill Livingstone. ISBN: 0443064229

Accident and Emergency Theory into Practice. Brian Dolan & Lynda Holt. Paperback 578 Pages 50 Illustrations (November 1999). Baillière Tindall. ISBN: 070202239X

Practical Procedures in the Emergency Department. John Bache. Paperback 176 Pages 297 Illustrations (July 1998). Mosby Wolfe Published. ISBN: 0723430136

References

Chapter 1

Code of Professional Conduct. United Kingdom Central Council for Nursing, Midwifery and Health Visiting. Original text document June 1992 (subsequently the Nursing and Midwifery Council (NMC).

Guidelines for the Administration of medicines. United Kingdom Central Council for Nursing, Midwifery and Health Visiting. Original text document October 2000 (subsequently the Nursing and Midwifery Council (NMC).

Guidelines for records and record keeping. United Kingdom Central Council for Nursing, Midwifery and Health Visiting. Original text document October 2000 (subsequently the Nursing and Midwifery Council (NMC).

Art & Science. Sept 18, vol 10, no. 52/1996. McColl E, Thomas L, Bond S (1996) A study to determine patient satisfaction with nursing care. *Nursing Standard*. 10, 52, 34–38. A study to determine patient satisfaction with nursing care

Journal of Advanced Nursing 29(1), 201–7, Blackwell Science Ltd.

Mentorship in nursing: a literature review, Margaret Andrews, BSc MSc RGN RCNT RNT[1] and Martha Wallis, BN(Hons) RGN RCNT RNT[2]

Chapter 2

Stress in an Accident and Emergency Department. *Irish Medical Journal*, March/April 2000, vol. 93, no. 2.

Struggling with Stress in Accident & Emergency. Irish Nurses Association. 14 August 2001 internet.

When waiting turns to anger in A&E, Audrey Gillan July 28, 2000, *The Guardian*, Society, Guardian.co.uk Guardian Newspapers Limited 2001.

Trauma Management vs. Stress Debriefing: What Should Responsible Organisations Do? Dr Jo Rick, Institute for Employment Studies, Brighton. Dr Rob Briner, Birkbeck College, University of London.

Chapter 3

Anatomical orientation, Biological Sciences Module Level 1 BSc.(Hons) Richard Collier, *http://www.sohp.soton.ac.uk/biosci/anatomy2.htm*

Update in Anaesthesia, Practical Procedures issue 6 (1996) Article 2, The management of trauma (Cont).

Nursing Research initiative for Scotland (NRIS) Newsletter vol. 11 March 2001.

An Investigation into Different Types of Thermometer for Measuring Temperature. Dawn Dowding (NRIS), Sarah Stevenson, Infection Control Nurse, Forth Valley Acute NHS Trust and members of the research group at Forth Valley Acute NHS Trust.

Physio.net. 1999 Physiotherapy Web Services. *http://www.physiotherapy.net.au/info/glossary/anaterms.htm*

Chapter 4

Management of Fingerip Injuries, Ravi Chittoria*, Swaran Arora** *Lecturer; **Prof and Head; Dept. of Plastic Surgery, Grant Medical College and Sir JJ Group of Hospitals, Mumbai 400 008. *http://www.bhj.org/journal/1999_4101_jan99/original_127.htm*

eMedicine Consumer Journal, July 6 2001, Volume 2, Number 7 (2001), eMedicine.com, Inc. Chad D Tarr, MD, Staff Physician, Department of Emergency Medicine, Emory University School of Medicine

Accident & emergency nursing. Rotator cuff injuries *R. H. Crusher* pp. 129–133, Volume 8, Number 3, July 2000.

Chapter 5

International Society for Arthroscopy knees Surgery and Orthopaedic Sports medicine. Healing of Soft Tissue: Time Constraints. William Stanish M.D., F.R.C.S.(C), F.A.C.S. Professor of Surgery, Dalhousie University Halifax, Nova Scotia, CANADA

A case-control study of the transit times through an Accident and Emergency department of ankle injured patients assessed using the Ottawa Ankle Rules. Vol. 8, Issue 3, July 2000, pp. 148–154. J. Allerston, D. Justham.

Chapter 6

Interventions for treating proximal humeral fractures in adults (Cochrane Review). Gibson JNA, Handoll HHG, Madhok R

Archives of family medicine, Vol. 9 No. 8, August 2000.

Management of Nasal Fractures, Brian Rubinstein, MD, MS; E. Bradley Strong, MD.

Canadian journal of surgery. Closed tibial shaft fractures: management and treatment complications. A review of the prospective literature. Chad P. Coles, MD; Michael Gross, MD. *Can J Surg* 2000, 43: 256–62.

Chapter 7

Accident & Emergency Nursing. Wound glue: a comparative study of tissue adhesives. A. Charters. pp. 223–227, Vol. 8, No. 4, October 2000.

Chapter 8

Myocardial infarction. The internet pathology laboratory web path. *http://www.nursing.about.com*

Congestive Heart Failure. Dondee Almazan, Sean McFarland, Lyza Sanders. California State University, Fresno Department of Nursing, Fresno, CA. *http://www.nursing.about.com*

Chapter 9

European Trauma Care Course. Thoracic Trauma. *http://www.trauma.org/eates/ectc/ectc-thorax.html*

6th Internet World Congress for Biomedical Sciences. Advances and Controversies in Acute Pain Management. Pain Management in Trauma Patients. Aldo Glik

Chapter 10

Outlines in Clinical Medicine. Abdominal Pain Differential, Jun 28, 1997. *http://www.geocities.com/Vienna/Studio/5466/OCM/difdx/4849.htm*

Chapter 11

Children Act 1989. 1989 Chapter 41. Crown Copyright 1989.

Chapter 12

Singapore Med J 1999, Vol. 40(05). What You Need To Know – Assessment of Suicide Risk, Y M Lai, S M Ko.

Web Sites for Nurses

One-minute summary – The internet, or world wide web, is an amazingly useful resource, giving the junior nurse huge amounts of information on any topic. Ignore this vast and valuable store of materials at your peril! Please note that neither the author nor the publisher are responsible for the content of the sites listed, which are simply intended to offer starting points for junior nurses. Also, please remember that the internet is a fast-evolving environment, and links may come and go. If you have some favourite sites you would like to see mentioned in future editions of this book, please write to Frank Durning, c/o Studymates (address on back cover). You will find a free readymade selection of nursing links at the Studymates web site:

httpı//www.studymates.co.uk

Happy surfing!

Web sites

Nursing & Midwifery Council
http://www.nmc-uk.org
Regulatory body for all registered nurses, midwives and health visitors in the UK.

British Journal of Nursing
http://www.markallengroup.com/bjn.htm
On this site you can find details of editorials, articles, courses, conferences and recruitment.

Care of the Emergency Patient (Course)
http://nursing.swan.ac.uk/d27.htm
Gives details of a diploma course covering the initial nursing assessment and management of patients who are present as a result of injury or acute illness. The course is run by the School of Health Science, the University of Wales, Swansea UK.

Clinical Links Site
http://www.damienvanc.ndirect.co.uk/
A growing clinical links site featuring hundreds of emergency care links.

CINAHL
http://www.cinahl.com/
The CINAHL database provides access to nursing and allied health literature and information from 1982 to the present. It covers virtually every nursing journal published, plus health topics such as physical therapy, occupational therapy, and emergency services, along with consumer health, and alternative therapies.

Cyber-Nurse
http://www.cyber-nurse.com/
Here's something a bit different looking – 'The Intergalactic Nurse's Station. Please allow our ancillary robots to be your guide while you are visiting!' A feature of Cyber-Nurse is its interactive question and answer section. Here you can view questions that other people have asked, or ask a question yourself.

Department of Health
http://www.doh.gov.uk/about.htm
The official web site of the UK Department of Health.

Emergency-Nurse
http://www.emergency-nurse.com/
Meeting a clear need, Emergency Nurse is the first online resource site for A&E nurses in the United Kingdom and overseas. It is run by nurses, for nurses. You are invited to contact the site if you would like to contribute to the body of information it is providing. The site maintains a directory of UK A&E nurses, ER nurses world wide, and others interested in the field of emergency nursing. View the latest pay scales, check out courses, conferences, the bookshop, articles, humour, email and more.

Emergency Nurses Association
http://www.ena.org
ENA's mission is to provide visionary leadership for emergency nursing and emergency care.

Emergency Nursing World (1)
http://ENW.org
A centre for clinical practice and informational needs of emergency nurses.

Emergency Nursing World (2)
http://www.hooked.net/~ttrimble/enw/index.html
A comprehensive site which contains articles, tips & tricks, links and much more.

Inter Nurse
http://www.internurse.com/
Internurse aims to be a nursing magazine on the internet, and more than just a links page. It aims to create the sort of nursing journal with all kinds of content, editorial, poetry, e-pals, support groups, bookstore, announce your own pages, professional information and links and more.

Journal of Emergency Medicine
http://www.bmjpg.com/data/aem.htm
This is a leading international journal of developments and advances in emergency medicine. Published by the *British Medical Journal* group, it represents all aspects of emergency care in both the hospital and pre-hospital environment. It acts as a forum for education, research, and debate on all aspects of emergency medicine. The site includes review articles, short reports, case reports and information on specific aspects of emergency care.

Medscape
http://www.medscape.com/
Medscape is a leading interactive web site for physicians, surgeons, nurses and consumers. At this impressive and large site you will find thousands of articles and clinical resources of all kinds. It aims to provide healthcare professionals with timely and directly applicable clinical information, to make the task of information gathering simpler and less time consuming; and to offer a broad medical audience clinical information with the depth, breadth, and validity needed to improve the practice of medicine.

Miningco Nursing
http://nursing.miningco.com/mbody.htm
This large and well presented site offers an enormous amount of information and links for nurses in all fields of practice.

Miningco Sports Medicine
http://sportsmedicine.miningco.com/
Here is an excellent source of anatomy and physiology in sports injury. It contains net links to anatomy and physiology, athletic training, body composition, conditioning, news, ergogenic aids, exercise physiology, fitness evaluation, flexibility, high altitude training, injuries and injury prevention, journals, nutrition for sport, organisations, over-training, rehabilitation, shoulder injuries, sport medicine clinics, sport psychology, surgery, women's issues, and a vast amount more.

Nurse Practitioner UK
http://www.healthcentre.org.uk/np/
Chat, groups, courses, conferences, notes and queries, and more for the nurse practitioner.

Nursing and Health Care Resources on the Net
http://www.shef.ac.uk/~nhcon/
This is an impressive list of nursing and health care resources set up and maintained by Rod Ward, a lecturer at the School of Nursing and Midwifery, University of Sheffield. He has designed the site to help nurses and other health professionals link up with resources on the net.

Nursing Net
http://www.nursingnet.org/
Nursing Net's mission is to help further knowledge and understanding of nursing, and to provide a forum for medical professionals and students to obtain and disseminate information about nursing and medically related subjects. Though American-based it is a valuable gateway to nursing information.

Nursing Standard Online
http://www.nursing-standard.co.uk/
This web site offers a selection of articles and abstracts from the latest weekly issue of *Nursing Standard*. Further details on all of its journals, conferences and continuing education opportunities are available by clicking on the relevant icon or text.

Nurse-zine
http://www.wwnurse.com/Nurse-zine/
Nurse-zine is a free monthly nursing email newsletter published since 1996 by World Wide Nurse, an internet nursing directory.

Online Journal of Issues in Nursing
http://www.nursingworld.org/ojin/index.htm
This is a peer-reviewed publication, presenting a number of different views on selected nursing issues.

Online Medical Dictionary
http://www.graylab.ac.uk/omd/index.html
Never be stuck for the definition of a medical or nursing term again! The site is quick, easy and free to use.

Royal College of Nursing
http://www.rcn.org.uk/
This is the electronic home of RCN Online. With more than 310,000 members, the RCN is the world's largest professional union of nurses. Run by nurses for nurses, it campaigns on the part of the profession, and is a leading player in the development of nursing practice and standards of care. On its impressive web site you can find a large amount of information about nursing – careers, training, resources, library facilities, research, post-registration and postgraduate opportunities at the RCN Institute, and much more. You can also read *Nursing Standard Online*, said to be the

first ever weekly nursing journal to publish on the internet.

Spring Net
http://www.springnet.com/sn/students.htm
A large US-based resource site for nursing students.

UK Health Centre
http://www.healthcentre.org.uk/
A guide to UK medical information on the web, maintained by David Rayne, a rural general practitioner in North Yorkshire. The site contains over 3,000 health-related links.

Virtual ER (Emergency Room)
http://www.virtualer.com/
'Where emergency medicine meets the internet.' You can find out about emergency medicine tutorials and lots more.

Virtual Nurse
http://virtualnurse.com/
Hundreds of pages of nursing resources, thousands of health links, discussion of nursing topics, nurse chats, nurse homepages, nursing polls, and nurses communicating with nurses from all over the world.

Weekly Web Review in Emergency Medicine
http://www.wwrem.com

World Wide Nurse
http://www.wwnurse.com/
This is a large US-based gateway site, leading to nursing links all over the world. There are sections on student nursing, clinical information, pharmacy, searching medical and nursing resources, employment opportunities and many other features.

World Wide Wounds
http://www.smtl.co.uk/World-Wide-Wounds/
Sign up here to receive the free *World Wide Wounds* email newsletter. It will tell you lots about wound management, wound care and dressings on the internet. The information is published by the UK Surgical Materials Testing Laboratory.

Wound Care Educational Guide
http://www.medicaledu.com/wndguide.htm
The Wound Care Information Network claims to have over 300 visitors a day. It offers some wound care discussion forums, where you can enter the discussion room of your choice, and post messages, comments or questions. Then, you can return in a few days to see if anyone has replied! Recent

forums included pressure ulcers, venous leg ulcers, and other wound care topics.

Newsgroups

Type in the following names into your browser's address panel, just as you would a web site address (no 'http://www' needed).

news:misc.education.medical
news:alt.npractitioners
news:sci.med.nursing

Index